AF711737

theclinics.com

CLINICS IN SPORTS MEDICINE

Sports Nutrition Update

GUEST EDITOR
Leslie Bonci, MPH, RD, LDN, CSSD

CONSULTING EDITOR
Mark D. Miller, MD

January 2007 • Volume 26 • Number 1

SAUNDERS
An Imprint of Elsevier, Inc.
PHILADELPHIA LONDON TORONTO MONTREAL SYDNEY TOKYO

W.B. SAUNDERS COMPANY
A Division of Elsevier Inc.

1600 John F. Kennedy Blvd. • Suite 1800 • Philadelphia, Pennsylvania 19103

http://www.theclinics.com

CLINICS IN SPORTS MEDICINE
January 2007
Editor: Debora Dellapena

Volume 26, Number 1
ISSN 0278-5919
ISBN-13: 978-1-4160-4296-9
ISBN-10: 1-4160-4296-2

Copyright © 2007 by Elsevier Inc. All rights reserved. No part of this publication may be reproduced or transmitted in any form or by any means, electronic or mechanical, including photocopy, recording, or any information retrieval system, without written permission from the Publisher.

Single photocopies of single articles may be made for personal use as allowed by national copyright laws. Permission of the publisher and payment of a fee is required for all other photocopying, including multiple or systematic copying, copying for advertising or promotional purposes, resale, and all forms of document delivery. Special rates are available for educational institutions that wish to make photocopies for non-profit educational classroom use. Permissions may be sought directly from Elsevier's Rights Department in Philadelphia, PA, USA: phone (+1) 215 239 3804, fax (+1) 215 239 3805, e-mail healthpermissions@elsevier.com. Requests may also be completed on-line via the Elsevier homepage (http://www.elsevier.com/locate/permissions). In the USA, users may clear permissions and make payments through the Copyright Clearance Center, Inc., 222 Rosewood Drive, Danvers, MA 01923, USA; phone: (978) 750-8400; fax: (978) 750-4744, and in the UK through the Copyright Licensing Agency Rapid Clearance Service (CLARCS), 90 Tottenham Court Road, London WIP 0LP, UK; phone (+44) 171 436 5931; fax: (+44) 171 436 3986. Other countries may have a local reprographic rights agency for payments.

Reprints: For copies of 100 or more, of articles in this publication, please contact the Commercial Reprints Department, Elsevier Inc., 360 Park Avenue South, New York, New York 10010-1710. Tel. (212) 633-3813; Fax: (212) 462-1935 e-mail: reprints@elsevier.com.

The ideas and opinions expressed in *Clinics in Sports Medicine* do not necessarily reflect those of the Publisher. The Publisher does not assume any responsibility for any injury and/or damage to persons or property arising out of or related to any use of the material contained in this periodical. The reader is advised to check the appropriate medical literature and the product information currently provided by the manufacturer of each drug to be administered to verify the dosage, the method and duration of administration, or contraindications. It is the responsibility of the treating physician or other health care professional, relying on independent experience and knowledge of the patient, to determine drug dosages and the best treatment for the patient. Mention of any product in this issue should not be construed as endorsement by the contributors, editors, or the Publisher of the product or manufacturers' claims.

Clinics in Sports Medicine (ISSN 0278-5919) is published quarterly by Elsevier Inc., 360 Park Avenue South, New York, NY 10010-1710. Months of publication are January, April, July, and October. Business and Editorial Offices: 1600 John F. Kennedy Blvd., Suite 1800, Philadelphia, PA 19103-2899. Customer Service Offices: 6277 Sea Harbor Drive, Orlando, FL 32887-4800. Periodicals postage paid at New York, NY, and additional mailing offices. Subscription prices are $205.00 per year (US individuals), $313.00 per year (US institutions), $103.00 per year (US students), $232.00 per year (Canadian individuals), $371.00 per year (Canadian institutions), $135.00 (Canadian students), $265.00 per year (foreign individuals), $371.00 per year (foreign institutions), and $135.00 per year (foreign students). Foreign air speed delivery is included in all *Clinics* subscription prices. All prices are subject to change without notice. POSTMASTER: Send address changes to *Clinics in Sports Medicine*, Elsevier Periodicals Customer Service, 6277 Sea Harbor Drive, Orlando, FL 32887-4800. **Customer Service: 1-800-654-2452 (US). From outside of the US, call 1-407-345-4000.** E-mail: hhspcs@harcourt.com.

Clinics in Sports Medicine is covered in *Index Medicus, Current Contents/Clinical Medicine, Excerpta Medica,* and *ISI/Biomed.*

Printed in the United States of America.

ELSEVIER
SAUNDERS

CLINICS IN SPORTS MEDICINE

Sports Nutrition Update

CONSULTING EDITOR

MARK D. MILLER, MD, Professor, Department of Orthopaedic Surgery; Head, Division of Sports Medicine, University of Virginia Health System, Charlottesville, Virginia

GUEST EDITOR

LESLIE BONCI, MPH, RD, LDN, CSSD, Director, Sports Medicine Nutrition, Department of Othopedic Surgery, Center for Sports Medicine, University of Pittsburgh Medical Center, Pittsburgh, Pennsylvania

CONTRIBUTORS

LAWRENCE E. ARMSTRONG, PhD, FACSM, Professor, Human Performance Laboratory, Department of Kinesiology, University of Connecticut, Storrs, Connecticut

KATHERINE A. BEALS, PhD, RD, FACSM, Clinical Associate Professor, Division of Nutrition and Department of Family and Preventive Medicine, University of Utah, Salt Lake City, Utah

DOUGLAS J. CASA, PhD, ATC, FACSM, Associate Professor, Human Performance Laboratory, Department of Kinesiology, University of Connecticut, Storrs, Connecticut

KRISTINE L. CLARK, PhD, RD, FACSM, Director of Sports Nutrition, Assistant Professor, Pennsylvania State University, University Park, Pennsylvania

ANN DUNAWAY, Graduate Student, Division of Nutrition, Georgia State University, Atlanta, Georgia

MATTHEW S. GANIO, MS, Doctoral Research Assistant, Human Performance Laboratory, Department of Kinesiology, University of Connecticut, Storrs, Connecticut

ROBERT M. MALINA, PhD, FACSM, Research Professor, Tarleton State University, Stephenville, Texas

CARL M. MARESH, PhD, FACSM, Professor and Head, Human Performance Laboratory, Department of Kinesiology, University of Connecticut, Storrs, Connecticut

NANNA L. MEYER, PhD, RD, Adjunct Assistant Professor, Division of Nutrition, University of Utah; and The Orthopedic Specialty Hospital (TOSH Sport Science), Salt Lake City, Utah

CHRISTINE A. ROSENBLOOM, PhD, RD, Professor, Division of Nutrition, Georgia State University, Atlanta, Georgia

KEVIN D. TIPTON, PhD, School of Sport and Exercise Sciences, University of Birmingham, Birmingham, United Kingdom

STELLA LUCIA VOLPE, PhD, RD, LDN, FACSM, Associate Professor and Miriam Stirl Term Endowed Chair of Nutrition, Division of Biobehavioral and Health Sciences, School of Nursing, University of Pennsylvania, Philadelphia, Pennsylvania

OLIVER C. WITARD, MSc, School of Sport and Exercise Sciences, University of Birmingham, Birmingham, United Kingdom

ELSEVIER
SAUNDERS

CLINICS IN SPORTS MEDICINE

Sports Nutrition Update

CONTENTS VOLUME 26 • NUMBER 1 • JANUARY 2007

ELSEVIER
SAUNDERS

CLINICS IN SPORTS MEDICINE

FORTHCOMING ISSUES

April 2007

Working as a Team Physician
Jeff G. Konin, PhD, ATC, PT
Guest Editor

July 2007

Infectious Disease and Sports Medicine
Tom Best, MD, PhD, and Jim Borchers, MD
Guest Editors

October 2007

ACL Graft and Fixation Choices
Jon K. Sekiya, MD, and Stephen B. Cohen, MD
Guest Editors

RECENT ISSUES

October 2006

Imaging of Lower Extremities
Timothy G. Sanders, MD
Guest Editor

July 2006

Imaging of Upper Extremities
Timothy G. Sanders, MD
Guest Editor

April 2006

Hip Injuries
Srino Bharam, MD, and
Marc J. Philippon, MD
Guest Editors

THE CLINICS ARE NOW AVAILABLE ONLINE!

Access your subscription at:
http://www.theclinics.com

Clin Sports Med 26 (2007) ix

CLINICS IN SPORTS MEDICINE

Foreword

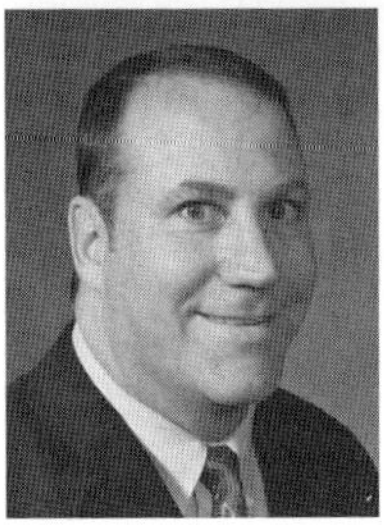

Mark D. Miller, MD

Consulting Editor

Here is an issue that is sure to whet your appetite–sports nutrition! Ever wonder how to plan a pregame meal or how to encourage your athletes to eat and drink the right stuff? Whatever happened to the female athlete triad–and does it just apply to anorexics? How about the "freshman 15"–does it apply to athletes? How about supplements? Are we making sure our athletes eat right? Is there any truth to the axiom that you are what you eat? Well, if you don't know–read on!

Mark D. Miller, MD
Department of Orthopaedic Surgery
Division of Sports Medicine
University of Virginia Health System
PO Box 800753
Charlottesville, VA 22903-0753, USA

E-mail address: mdm3p@hscmail.mcc.virginia.edu

0278-5919/07/$ – see front matter
doi:10.1016/j.csm.2006.11.007

© 2007 Elsevier Inc. All rights reserved.
sportsmed.theclinics.com

Clin Sports Med 26 (2007) xi–xii

CLINICS IN SPORTS MEDICINE

Preface

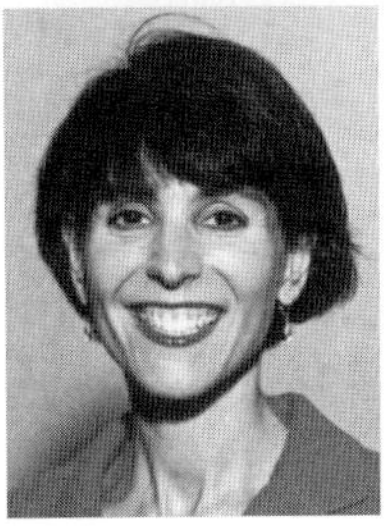

Leslie Bonci, MPH, RD, LDN, CSSD

Guest Editor

Sports nutrition is often the missing piece in the athlete's training regimen. The attention and effort are directed toward optimizing strength, speed, stamina, and recovery, but too often, nutrition is not the priority, resulting in performance impairment rather than enhancement. Sports medicine professionals need to be able to educate athletes on not only the what (food and drink), but also the why, when, where, and how much to consume. Athletes are bombarded with nutrition information, but much of what they read can be contradictory, confusing, or incorrect.

As important as hydration is to performance, most athletes fall short of recommendations. Ganio and colleagues provide a new look at this issue and put to rest some of the fallacies surrounding hydration.

Athletes know that carbohydrates are important to optimize performance and recovery, but there is a lot of controversy surrounding protein requirements. Tipton and Witard present the theoretical recommendations along with the practical so that we can more appropriately educate athletes.

Body composition is a sensitive but sometimes necessary issue to address with athletes, but incorrect standards may lead to deleterious consequences for athletes. Malina offers recommendations for body composition assessment and estimated body fat so that we can provide science-based tables to help athletes with body composition concerns.

Beals and Meyer share insight into some of the devastating consequences of the female athlete triad and how to manage an athlete who is affected by the triad.

Rosenbloom and Dunaway focus on nutritional recommendations for masters athletes, a rapidly growing field. Clark and Volpe address two other

0278-5919/07/$ – see front matter
doi:10.1016/j.csm.2006.11.008

© 2007 Elsevier Inc. All rights reserved.

"hot" areas: Nutrient recommendations for joint health and micronutrient requirements for athletes.

If we provide athletes with factual, practical, and science-based sports nutrition recommendations, we keep them in their game, optimize their health, and expedite their recovery from injury.

A round of applause to all the authors for their excellent and insightful contributions in providing food for thought, and to Deb Dellapena for bringing this edition to fruition.

Leslie Bonci, MPH, RD, LDN, CSSD
Sports Medicine Nutrition
Department of Othopedic Surgery
Center for Sports Medicine
University of Pittsburgh Medical Center
200 Lothrop Street, Pittsburgh, PA 15213-2582, USA

E-mail address: boncilj@upmc.edu

Clin Sports Med 26 (2007) 1–16

CLINICS IN SPORTS MEDICINE

ELSEVIER SAUNDERS

Evidence-Based Approach to Lingering Hydration Questions

Matthew S. Ganio, MS, Douglas J. Casa, PhD, ATC*, Lawrence E. Armstrong, PhD, Carl M. Maresh, PhD

Human Performance Laboratory, Department of Kinesiology, University of Connecticut, 2095 Hillside Road, U-1110, Storrs, CT 06269-1110, USA

Studies related to fundamental hydration issues have required clinicians to re-examine certain practices and concepts. The ingestion of substances such as creatine, caffeine, and glycerol has been questioned in regards to safety and hydration status. Reports of overdrinking (hyponatremia) also have brought into question the practices of drinking appropriate fluid amounts and the role that fluid-electrolyte balance has in the etiology of heat illnesses such as heat cramps. This article offers a fresh perspective on timely topics related to hydration, fluid balance, and exercise in the heat.

CORE TEMPERATURE AND HYDRATION

Proper hydration is important for optimal sport performance [1] and may play a role in the prevention of heat illnesses [2]. Dehydration increases cardiovascular strain and increases core temperature (T_c) to levels higher than in a state of euhydration [3]. These increases, independently [4] and in combination [3,5], impair performance and put an individual at risk for heat illness [6]. Exercise in the heat in which dehydration occurs before [3] or during exercise [7] results in T_c that is directly correlated ($r = 0.98$) [7] with degree of dehydration (Fig. 1). The link between dehydration and hyperthermia has shown that independently and additively they result in cardiovascular instability that puts individuals at risk for heat exhaustion [3].

Despite laboratory evidence linking dehydration with increased T_c, some authors argue that this physiologic phenomenon does not occur in field settings [8–10]. This may be because field studies fail to control exercise intensity [8–11]. T_c is driven by metabolic rate, and when the same subject is tested in a controlled laboratory environment, a higher metabolic rate produces a higher T_c [12]. Without controlling or measuring relative exercise intensity, a hydrated individual could exercise at a higher metabolic rate and drive his or her T_c to the same level as a dehydrated individual working at a lower intensity. Without

*Corresponding author. *E-mail address:* douglas.casa@uconn.edu (D.J. Casa).

0278-5919/07/$ – see front matter
doi:10.1016/j.csm.2006.11.001

© 2007 Elsevier Inc. All rights reserved.

sportsmed.theclinics.com

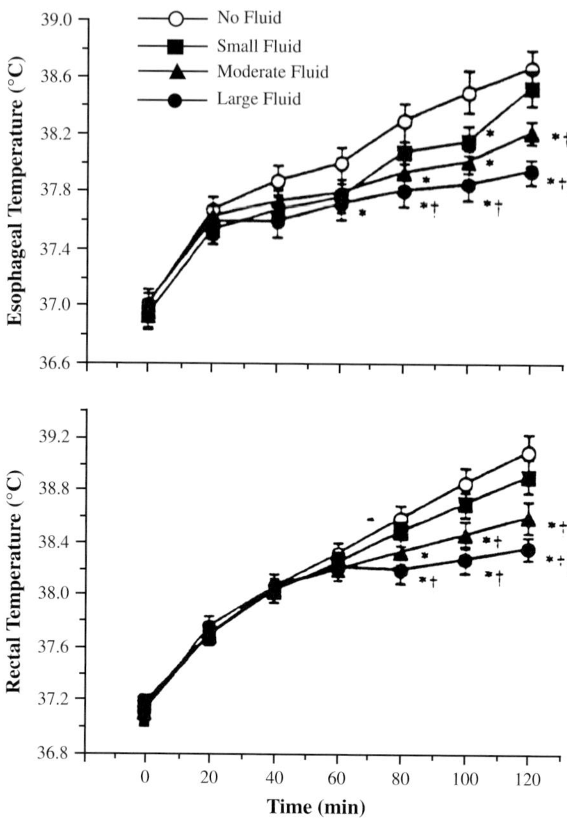

Fig. 1. The degree of dehydration that occurs during exercise is correlated with the increase in esophageal (*top graph*) and rectal (*bottom graph*) temperatures. Subjects cycled for 120 minutes in a 33°C environment at approximately 65% VO_{2max} while replacing 0% (No Fluid), 20% (Small Fluid), 48% (Moderate Fluid), or 81% (Large Fluid) of the fluid lost in sweat. Subjects lost 4.2%, 3.4%, 2.3%, and 1.1% body weight in the conditions. (*From* Montain SJ, Coyle EF. Influence of graded dehydration on hyperthermia and cardiovascular drift during exercise. J Appl Physiol 1992;73(4):1340–50; with permission.)

a randomized crossover experimental design that controls exercise intensity, field studies cannot validly conclude that hydration is not linked to T_c.

Field studies disputing relationships between T_c and dehydration also cite that laboratory studies use environments that are too hot, and that the physiologic relationship does not exist in temperate environments (approximately 23°C) often associated with field studies [8]. Laboratory studies have shown that the increase of T_c with dehydration is exacerbated in hot environments, but still observed in cold environments (8°C) [13]. Dehydration impairs thermoregulation independent of ambient conditions, but the effect is seen especially at high ambient temperatures when the thermoregulatory system is more heavily stressed. Laboratory-based studies have clearly shown that when exercise intensity and hydration state are controlled, T_c increases at a faster rate when subjects are dehydrated [7].

CAFFEINE

Caffeine and its related compounds, theophylline and theobromine, have long been recognized as diuretic molecules [14], which encourage excretion of urine via increased blood flow to the kidneys [15]. The recommendation that caffeine be avoided by athletes because hydration status would be compromised [6] is based on several studies examining the acute effects of high levels (>300 mg) of caffeine [16]. More recent studies have tested the credibility of this recommendation by re-examining hydration status in varying settings after short-term caffeine intake and, for the first time, after long-term intake.

Using increased urine output as an indicator of diuresis and dehydration, early studies showed that the threshold for an increase of urine output was 250 to 300 mg of caffeine intake [17]. Urine output was greater for the first 3 hours after ingestion [17], but when urine was collected for 4 hours, the difference in urine output between caffeine and placebo was negated [18]. When double the caffeine was ingested (612 mg or 8.5 mg/kg), urine volume increased over the next 4 hours [19]. The molecular properties of caffeine do not refute the fact that it may act as an acute diuretic, but when observations span a short time (<24 hours), it is difficult to understand long-term changes in hydration [15].

When 24-hour urine volume is examined, the ingestion of caffeine at levels of 1.4 to 3.1 mg/kg does not increase urine output or change hydration status [20]. When large amounts of caffeine are ingested (8.2–10.2 mg/kg), the increases in urine excretion vary from person to person, but may be 41% greater than control levels [21]. It cannot be concluded from these studies that "caffeine causes dehydration" because acute increases in urine volume with large caffeine intake (>300 mg) may be offset later by decreased urine output and result in no change in long-term hydration status [16].

Acute ingestion of caffeine before exercise (1–2 hours) at levels up to 8.7 mg/kg does not alter urine output and fluid balance [19,22–24] when subjects exercise at 60% to 85% VO_{2max} for 0.5 to 3 hours [19,22–24]. The possible mechanism for a lack of a diuretic effect with caffeine during exercise is most likely due to an increase in catecholamines and diminished renal blood flow [19]. There is little evidence to suggest that short-term use of caffeine alters hydration status at rest or during exercise.

Because most Americans consume caffeine on a regular basis [15], it is surprising that few studies have examined the effects of controlled caffeine intake over several days. In 2004, the authors' research team conducted a field study involving a crossover design in which subjects exercised for 2 hours, twice a day, for 3 consecutive days [25]. Subjects rehydrated ad libitum and consumed a volume equal to 7 cans daily of either caffeinated or decaffeinated soda. Throughout the 3 days, no differences of urine volume, body weight, plasma volume, and urine specific gravity were observed between the two conditions. The authors reported similar results in an investigation in which subjects consumed 3 mg caffeine/kg/d for 6 days; during the following 5 days, 20 subjects decreased their intake to 0 mg/kg/d, 20 maintained intake at 3 mg/kg/d, and 20 doubled their intake to 6 mg/kg/d [26]. Urine volume and other markers of hydration status showed that, regardless of caffeine ingestion, hydration status did not change throughout the 11 days (Fig. 2). Heat tolerance and thermoregulation examined on the 12th day during exercise in a hot environment did not differ between conditions [27].

Acute ingestion of moderate to low levels of caffeine (<300 mg) does not promote dehydration at rest or during exercise. Long-term ingestion of low to high levels of caffeine does not compromise hydration status and thermoregulation at rest and during exercise. Varying one's level of caffeine ingestion (either increasing or decreasing) also does not seem to change hydration status [15,16]. There is no evidence to support caffeine restriction on the basis of impaired thermoregulation or changes of hydration status at levels less than 300–400 mg/d.

HYPONATREMIA

Hyponatremia has received attention in the media as a result of its occurrence in popular road running races [28]. Hyponatremia is a serious complication of low plasma sodium levels (<130 mEq/L) [29]. The exact cause is likely multifaceted and circumstantial [30]. Hyponatremia has been observed in exercising individuals who became dehydrated [31,32], maintained hydration [32], and became overhydrated [31,32]. Asymptomatic hyponatremia is the most common type of hyponatremia [32] and is defined as a decrease in sodium level (<130 mEq/L) that occurs in the absence of life-threatening symptoms [33]. Asymptomatic hyponatremia per se is not harmful or detrimental to performance [34]. When plasma sodium decreases to less than 125 mEq/L, hyponatremic illness may occur. Hyponatremic illness is a medical emergency that is symptomatic and requires immediate medical treatment [32,33,35].

Overdrinking, identified as an increase in body mass, significantly increases one's risk for developing hyponatremia and should be avoided [32,35,36]. Some observational studies have found that increased dehydration results in higher sodium levels [31,32,37], but this does not mean that dehydration prevents hyponatremia. The increased risk of heat illnesses associated with dehydration does not warrant dehydration as a method for preventing hyponatremia. High sweat rates or sodium-concentrated sweat may lead to large losses of sodium and put one at risk for hyponatremia, especially in events lasting more than 3 hours [38]. It is recommended that one should ingest fluid at a rate that closely matches fluid loss (ie, ≤2% body weight loss) [39].

Replacing large fluid losses with equal amounts of pure water may dilute the plasma sodium level [36], so it has been suggested that replacement of electrolytes can be achieved through sports drinks or salt tablets [30,34]. Mathematical modeling has shown that in a variety of conditions the ingestion of sodium may attenuate the decline of serum sodium over time (Fig. 3) [40]. However, recent

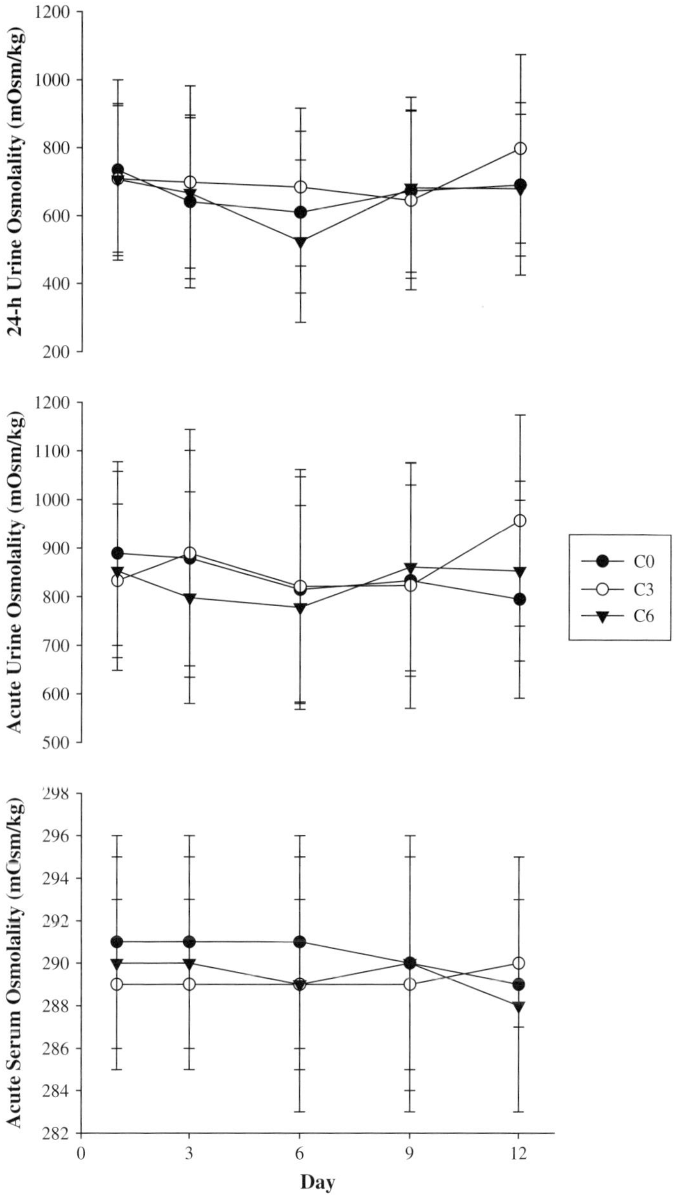

Fig. 2. Controlled consumption of caffeine at a level of 3 mg/kg/d for 6 days and then decreased to 0 mg/kg/d (C0), maintained at 3 mg/kg/d (C3), or increased to 6 mg/kg/d (C6); none of these conditions altered hydration status. Urine osmolality (*top graph*) and volume (data not shown) during repeated 24-hour collection periods did not change over the course of the investigation. Acute urine (*middle graph*) and serum (*bottom graph*) osmolality also did not differ as a result of the level of caffeine consumption. (*Data from* Armstrong LE, Pumerantz AC, Roti MW, et al. Fluid, electrolyte, and renal indices of hydration during 11 days of controlled caffeine consumption. Int J Sport Nutr Exerc Metab 2005;15(3):252–65.)

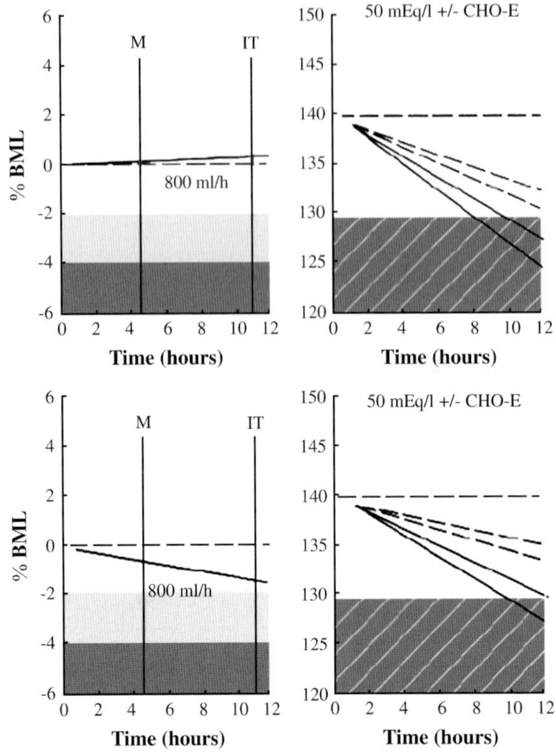

Fig. 3. Predicted effectiveness of a carbohydrate-electrolyte sports drink (CHO-E) containing 17 mEq/L of sodium and 5 mEq/L of potassium for attenuating the decline in plasma sodium concentration (mEq/L) expected for a 70-kg person drinking water at 800 mL/h when running 10 km/h in cool (18°C; *upper panel*) and warm (28°C; *lower panel*) environments. The solid shaded areas depict water loss that would be sufficient to diminish performance modestly and substantially. The hatched shaded area indicates the presence of hyponatremia. *M* indicates the finishing time for the marathon run. *IT* indicates the approximate finishing time for an iron-man triathlon. For the sodium figures, the solid lines reflect the effect of drinking water only, and hatched lines illustrate the effect of consuming the same volume of a sports drink. The pair of lines of similar type represent the predicated outcomes when total body water accounts for 50% and 63% of body mass. BML, body mass loss. (*From* Montain SJ, Cheuvront SN, Sawka MN. Exercise associated hyponatraemia: quantitative analysis to understand the etiology. Br J Sports Med 2006;40(2):98–105; with permission.)

studies involving consumption of sodium through sports drinks and salt tablets have confirmed [30,34,41] and refuted [37,42,43] this relationship (Fig. 4). Some of these differences in results may lie in methodologic differences, [30] assumptions, and conflicting conclusions [44].

Understanding the etiology and cause of hyponatremia may help to understand its prevention better. It is well agreed that overconsumption of fluids is the primary, but not the only, cause [35,40]. Whether replacement of sweat losses with equal volumes of sodium-containing beverages would prevent or

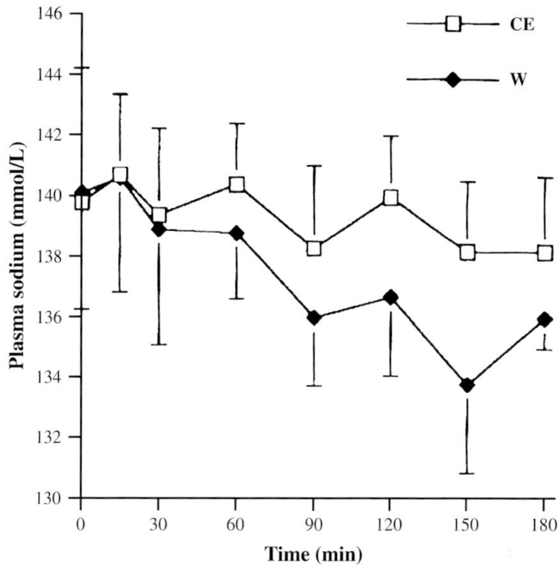

Fig. 4. Ingestion of a carbohydrate-electrolyte beverage (CE) slightly attenuated the decline of plasma sodium observed with ingestion of plain water (W) over 180 minutes of exercise at a moderate intensity in a hot environment (34°C). (*Adapted from* Vrijens DM, Rehrer NJ. Sodium-free fluid ingestion decreases plasma sodium during exercise in the heat. J Appl Physiol 1999;86(6):1847–51; with permission.)

attenuate hyponatremia is still debated [35]. More studies that look at varying environmental conditions, sweat rates, and body masses may help shed light on this complex picture. Some authorities have suggested that allowing dehydration would prevent hyponatremia because the contraction of extracellular fluid would increase sodium concentration. Until further studies are conducted, promoting dehydration (ie, >2% of pre-exercise weight) is not warranted and may put some individuals at greater risk for exertional heat illnesses and could compromise performance [2].

CREATINE

Creatine is one of the most popular nutritional supplements on the market. Athletes of all levels and varieties of sports are using it in hopes of gaining a competitive edge. During creatine supplementation, 90% of the increase in body weight (0.7–2.0 kg) is accounted for by increases of total body water (TBW) [45]. The increase of TBW during the "loading phase" results from increases of intracellular water stores [46], but prolonged use of creatine results in TBW increases in all body fluid compartments [45]. Some authors speculate that creatine use while exercising in the heat impairs heat tolerance and may be a contributing factor for heatstroke [47,48]. Those authors propose that creatine increases one's risk for heat injury because the increases of intracellular water stores deplete intravascular volume [49]. Before any published conclusive studies concerning creatine's effect on hydration status and use in the heat, the American College of Sports Medicine published a consensus statement stating that "high-dose creatine supplementation should be avoided during periods of increased thermal stress ... there are concerns about the possibility of altered fluid balance, and impaired sweating and thermoregulation ..." [48].

Paradoxically, studies using short-term and long-term creatine supplementation have shown that subjects exercising in the heat (30–37°C) for 80 minutes have either no change or an advantageous lower heart rate and T_c [46,50–52]. Work from our laboratory also has shown that creatine supplementation does not alter exercise heat tolerance, even when subjects begin exercise in a dehydrated state (Fig. 5) [51]. One study that found lower T_c with creatine use during exercise in heat suggests that the increases of TBW with supplementation may hyperhydrate the body and lower T_c [46]. Despite early concerns about creatine supplementation and exercise in the heat [48], more recent studies have shown conclusively that heat storage does not increase as a result of creatine use [46,50–52]. There is no evidence to support restriction of creatine use during exercise in the heat.

EXERCISE-ASSOCIATED CRAMPS

Although the exact mechanism is unknown, skeletal muscle cramps are associated with numerous congenital and acquired conditions, including hereditary

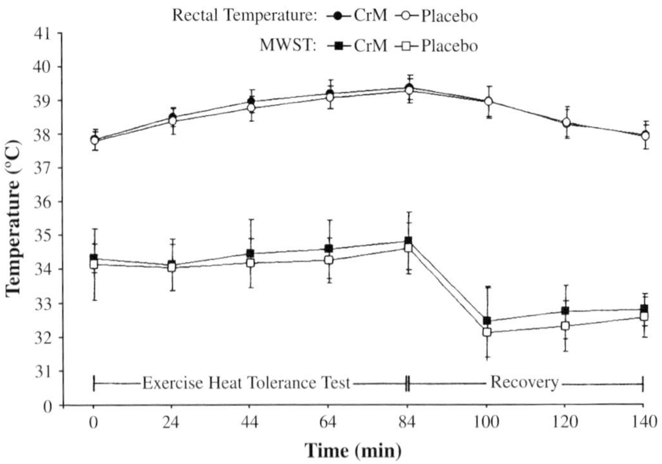

Fig. 5. The use of creatine monohydrate (CrM) does not compromise exercise heat tolerance. After becoming dehydrated, rectal temperature and mean weighted skin temperature (MWST) had similar responses in CrM and placebo treatments when subjects exercised in the heat and recovered in a cool environment. (*From* Watson G, Casa D, Fiala KA, et al. Creatine use and exercise heat tolerance in dehydrated men. J Athl Train 2006;41(1):18–29; with permission.)

disorders of carbohydrate and lipid metabolism, diseases of neuromuscular and endocrine origins, fluid and electrolyte deficits (ie, owing to diarrhea or vomiting), pharmacologic agents (ie, β-agonists, ethanol, diuretics), and toxins [53]. The medical treatments for these various forms of muscle cramps are as varied as their etiologies. McGee [54] specifically classified leg muscle cramps as contractures (ie, electrically silent cramps caused by myopathy or disease), tetany (ie, sensory plus motor unit hyperactivity), dystonia (ie, simultaneous contraction of agonist and antagonist muscles), or true cramps (ie, motor unit hyperactivity). The last category includes skeletal muscle cramps that are due to heat, fluid-electrolyte disturbances, hemodialysis, and medications.

The International Classification of Diseases [55] defines heat cramps, a form of motor unit hyperactivity, as painful involuntary contractions that are associated with large sweat (ie, water and sodium) losses. Heat cramps occur most often in active muscles (ie, thigh, calf, and abdominal) that have been challenged by a single prolonged event (ie, >2–4 hours) or during consecutive days of physical exertion. A high incidence of heat cramps occurs among tennis players [56], American football players [57], steel mill workers [58], and soldiers who deploy to hot environments [59,60]. These activities result in a large sweat loss, consumption of hypotonic fluid or pure water, and a whole-body sodium and water imbalance [59,61]. The distinctions between heat cramps and other forms of exercise-associated cramps are subtle [54,59,62], but sodium replacement usually resolves heat cramps effectively [56,59,61–63]; successful treatment via sodium administration confirms a preliminary diagnosis of heat cramps.

Bergeron [62] described a tennis player who was plagued by recurring heat cramps. This athlete secreted sweat at a rate of 2.5 L/h and had a sweat sodium (Na^+) concentration of 83 mEq/L. This sweat Na^+ concentration is high, in that most heat-acclimatized athletes exhibit 20 to 40 mEq Na^+/L of sweat (ie, heat acclimatization reduces sweat Na^+ concentration), but occurs naturally in a small percentage of humans. During 4 hours of tennis match play, this young athlete lost 10 L of sweat and a large quantity of electrolytes (ie, 830 mEq of Na^+; 19,090 mg of Na^+; 48.6 g of sodium chloride). Given that the average sodium chloride intake of adults in the United States is 8.7 g (3.4 g Na^+) per day, it is not difficult to see how this athlete could experience a whole-body Na^+ deficit. To offset his 4-hour sodium chloride loss in sweat, this athlete would require 1.6 L of normal saline, 7.8 to 9.8 cans of canned soup (85–107 mEq per can), 12.6 servings of tomato juice (66 mEq of Na^+ per serving), or 39.5 to 127.7 L of a sport drink (6.5–21 mEq Na^+/L). These options are unreasonable. A long history of heat cramps ended when this tennis player began consuming supplemental salt during meals. Other tennis players have been successfully treated using a similar course of action [63].

In 2004, the authors' research team evaluated a female varsity basketball player (body mass 78.5 kg, height 187 cm) who experienced exercise-induced cramps during the winter months in New England, with signs and symptoms identical to heat cramps. The authors measured her sweat rate as 1.16 L/h, her sweat sodium concentration (ie, via whole-body washdown) as 42 mEq/L, and her daily consumption of sodium. These values were normal and typical of winter sport athletes. Three days of observations indicated that her dietary intake of Na^+ per day was similar to her daily sweat Na^+ loss (ie, both 3200–3600 mg). Because she did not train or compete in a hot environment, the authors hesitated to diagnose her malady as heat cramps. When she began ingesting supplemental sodium (ie, by liberally salting each meal at midseason), however, the skeletal muscle cramps resolved permanently. This case suggests that a history of skeletal muscle cramps, with a large daily Na^+ turnover owing to a high sweat rate, indicates the need for an evaluation of whole-body Na^+ balance. It further suggests that heat cramps may have been named because they usually occur in hot environments, but they also may occur in mild environments when sweat Na^+ concentration and sweat losses are large.

A study by Stofan and colleagues [57] examined the link between sweat sodium losses and heat cramps. Sweat rate, sodium content, and percent body weight loss were measured on a single day of a "two-a-day" practice in subjects who had a history (episode within the last year) of severe heat cramps. Although heat cramps were not observed, football players with a history of heat cramps had sweat sodium losses two times greater than matched controls. Although the exact etiology of heat cramps may be unknown, sodium deficits seem to contribute to their development. In most cases, restoration and compensation of sodium losses seems to prevent further heat cramps.

FLUID NEEDS AND HYDRATION PLAN

Water losses during exercise should be replaced at a rate equal to (not greater than) the sweat rate [39]. Loss of sweat during exercise needs to be replaced after exercise, but dehydration ($\geq$2% body weight) during exercise can be detrimental to performance in part by increases in T_c. It is difficult to replace 100% of fluid loss during exercise, especially if it occurs in hot environments for long durations or if sweat loss is great [11,39]. Authorities have suggested that a minimal amount of dehydration (<2% body weight) may be tolerated without compromising performance [64]. Regardless, knowledge of sweat rate is necessary to develop a hydration plan (Table 1) [65], but without this it has been recommended to ingest 200 to 300 mL every 10 to 20 minutes [6]. Thirst lags behind changes in hydration (termed *voluntary dehydration*) [66]. When individuals have high sweat rates, and large volumes of fluid cause gastrointestinal stress, it may be advantageous for them to train themselves to tolerate consumption of fluids at a rate similar to their sweat losses [67].

In attempts to optimize endurance performance in the heat, glycerol has been used to increase TBW. It is an osmotically active molecule that acutely (<4 hours) increases TBW stores [68]. Although using glycerol plus water is an effective prehydration strategy, it does not increase sweat rate or reduce performance time or T_c in a race setting [69]. Using glycerol as a part of a rehydration strategy between exercise bouts increases exercise time to exhaustion in the heat (37°C). The increase is likely due to increases of plasma volume, not because of cardiovascular effects, thermoregulatory effects, or differences in fluid-regulating hormones [70]. It is generally accepted that glycerol, although a hyperhydrating agent, is not an ergogenic aid in most situations [64]. Future research should examine the importance of timing in glycerol ingestion for performance benefits.

When multiple, dehydrating exercise sessions are occurring over a short time (ie, two workouts per day in football or track and field), athletes must rehydrate immediately and quickly between bouts. Intravenous rehydration has been used in the belief that direct administration of fluid into the central circulation optimally replaces lost fluid. Contrary to this belief, when hydrating with equal amounts of intravenous and oral fluid ingestion, intravenous is not superior to restore plasma volume after dehydration [71]. Oral rehydration results in better cardiovascular stability, lower T_c, rating of perceived exertion, thirst, and thermal sensation than intravenous rehydration. However, these changes do not translate into improved exercise time to exhaustion [71,72]. Regardless, oral hydration is preferred (versus intravenous) for individuals who would be exercising subsequently in the heat [71,72]. An exception occurs when large amounts of fluid must be replaced in a short time, and gastric emptying and intestinal absorption rates may limit the ingestion of fluids orally. In such cases, a combination of intravenous and oral rehydration may be warranted so that fluid requirements are met, and the oropharyngeal reflex is stimulated [73].

Athletes often supplement with glycerol or choose to use intravenous rehydration because of the difficulty of matching fluid intake with fluid losses during intense exercise in the heat. This makes theoretical sense given the possibility of large sweat rates (ie, >1.5 L/h) and the likelihood that fluid consumption could not match the sweat rate given gastric emptying and intestinal absorption rates, especially when the ingestion must occur when the exercise is intense. An individualized rehydration plan that considers sweat rate, the semantics of the actual competition parameters, and personal preferences and tolerance is recommended to ensure that rehydration is optimized in these circumstances [65]. When the individualized rehydration plan is practiced and rehearsed in practices and preliminary competitions, the need for glycerol and intravenous rehydration will likely be eliminated because of the benefits associated with the "rehydration training," and ultimately the degree of dehydration would be minimized [65,74].

SUMMARY

Hydration status affects exercise performance in the heat and may influence the development of exertional heat illnesses. However, numerous factors that influence hydration state are not understood by the public. Field-based studies may lead athletes to believe that T_c is not influenced by hydration, but these studies contradict well-controlled laboratory experiments. For many years, recommendations have been published that active individuals should avoid caffeinated

Table 1
Self-testing program for optimal hydration*

1. Make sure you are properly hydrated *before* the workout—your urine should be pale yellow
2. Do a warmup run until you begin to sweat, then stop. Urinate if necessary
3. Weigh yourself naked on a floor scale (accurate to 0.1 kg)
4. Run for 1 h at an intensity similar to your targeted race or training run
5. Drink a measured amount of a beverage during the run, if you are thirsty. It is important that you measure exactly how much fluid you consume during the run
6. Do not urinate until post-body weight is recorded
7. Weigh yourself naked again on the same scale you used in step 3
8. You may now urinate and drink fluids as needed. Calculate your fluid need using the following formula

A. Enter your body weight from step 3 in Kg (To convert from lb to kg, divide lb by 2.2)		________
B. Enter your body weight from step 7 in Kg (To convert from lb to kg, divide lb by 2.2)		________
C. Subtract B from A	A–B =	________
D. Convert your total in step C to g by multiplying by 1000	C × 1000 =	________
E. Enter the amount of fluid consumed during the run in mL (To convert from oz to mL, multiply oz by 30)		________
F. Add E to D	E + D =	________

This final figure is the number of ml that you need to consume per hour to remain well hydrated. If you want to convert mL back to oz, divide by 30

*This table may be used to calculate the amount of fluid needed during an exercise bout to remain hydrated.

Adapted from Casa D. Proper hydration for distance running—identifying individual fluid needs. Track Coach 2004;167:5321–8; with permission.

beverages with little supporting scientific evidence. Research from the authors' laboratory shows that long-term intake of moderate levels of caffeine does not compromise hydration status. Hyponatremia also has received a lot of attention, but until more is known about its etiology and prevention, it is recommended that athletes drink an amount of fluid to minimize dehydration (but not overdrink). The use of creatine as an ergogenic aid initially was overshadowed by questions regarding its safety during exercise in the heat. Research shows no reason for these concerns. Although the mechanism of heat cramps is still not fully understood, it seems that deficits in sodium from sweating and/or diet is a predisposing factor. The reader is encouraged to read thorough review articles on these topics [64,75]. Ultimately, clinical practice should be dictated by evidence in the literature and not perpetuate unproven myths.

References

[1] Armstrong LE, Costill DL, Fink WJ. Influence of diuretic-induced dehydration on competitive running performance. Med Sci Sports Exerc 1985;17(4):456–61.

[2] Binkley HM, Beckett J, Casa DJ, et al. National Athletic Trainers' Association position statement: exertional heat illnesses. J Athl Train 2002;37(3):329–43.
[3] Gonzalez-Alonso J, Mora-Rodriguezk R, Below PR, et al. Dehydration markedly impairs cardiovascular function in hyperthermic endurance athletes during exercise. J Appl Physiol 1997;82(4):1229–36.
[4] Gonzalez-Alonso J, Teller C, Andersen SL, et al. Influence of body temperature on the development of fatigue during prolonged exercise in the heat. J Appl Physiol 1999;86(3): 1032–9.
[5] Gonzalez-Alonso J. Separate and combined influences of dehydration and hyperthermia on cardiovascular responses to exercise. Int J Sports Med 1998;19(Suppl 2):S111–4.
[6] Casa DJ, Armstrong LE, Hillman SK, et al. National Athletic Trainers' Association position statement: fluid replacement for athletes. J Athl Train 2000;35(2):212–24.
[7] Montain SJ, Coyle EF. Influence of graded dehydration on hyperthermia and cardiovascular drift during exercise. J Appl Physiol 1992;73(4):1340–50.
[8] Laursen PB, Suriano R, Quod MJ, et al. Core temperature and hydration status during an ironman triathlon. Br J Sports Med 2006;40(4):320–5.
[9] Godek SF, Bartolozzi AR, Burkholder R, et al. Core temperature and percentage of dehydration in professional football linemen and backs during preseason practices. J Athl Train 2006;41(1):8–17.
[10] Sharwood KA, Collins M, Goedecke JH, et al. Weight changes, medical complications, and performance during an ironman triathlon. Br J Sports Med 2004;38(6):718–24.
[11] Godek SF, Godek JJ, Bartolozzi AR. Hydration status in college football players during consecutive days of twice-a-day preseason practices. Am J Sports Med 2005;33:843–51.
[12] Sawka MN, Wenger CB. Physiological responses to acute exercise-heat stress. In: Pandolf KB, Sawka MN, Gonzalez RR, editors. Human performance physiology and environmental medicine at terrestrial extremes. Traverse City: Cooper Publishing Group; 1988. p. 97–151.
[13] Gonzalez-Alonso J, Mora-Rodriguez R, Coyle EF. Stroke volume during exercise: interaction of environment and hydration. Am J Physiol Heart Circ Physiol 2000;278(2):H321–30.
[14] Eddy NB, Downs AW. Tolerance and cross-tolerance in the human subject to the diuretic effect of caffeine, theobromine, and theophylline. J Pharmacol Exp Ther 1928;33:167–74.
[15] Armstrong LE. Caffeine, body fluid electrolyte balance, and exercise performance. Int J Sport Nutr Exerc Metab 2002;12(2):189–206.
[16] Maughan RJ, Griffin J. Caffeine ingestion and fluid balance: a review. J Hum Nutr Dietet 2003;16:411–20.
[17] Robertson D, Frolich JC, Carr RK, et al. Effects of caffeine on plasma renin activity, catecholamines and blood pressure. N Engl J Med 1978;298(4):181–6.
[18] Passmore AP, Kondowe GB, Johnston GD. Renal and cardiovascular effects of caffeine: a dose-response study. Clin Sci (Lond) 1987;72(6):749–56.
[19] Wemple RD, Lamb DR, McKeever KH. Caffeine vs caffeine-free sports drinks: effects on urine production at rest and during prolonged exercise. Int J Sports Med 1997;18(1):40–6.
[20] Grandjean AC, Reimers KJ, Bannick KE, et al. The effect of caffeinated, non-caffeinated, caloric and non-caloric beverages on hydration. J Am Coll Nutr 2000;19(5):591–600.
[21] Neuhauser B, Beine S, Verwied SC, et al. Coffee consumption and total body water homeostasis as measured by fluid balance and bioelectrical impedance analysis. Ann Nutr Metab 1997;41(1):29–36.
[22] Graham TE, Hibbert E, Sathasivam P. Metabolic and exercise endurance effects of coffee and caffeine ingestion. J Appl Physiol 1998;85(3):883–9.
[23] Falk B, Burstein R, Rosenblum J, et al. Effects of caffeine ingestion on body fluid balance and thermoregulation during exercise. Can J Physiol Pharmacol 1990;68(7):889–92.
[24] Gordon NF, Myburgh JL, Kruger PE, et al. Effects of caffeine ingestion on thermoregulatory and myocardial function during endurance performance. S Afr Med J 1982;62(18): 644–7.

[25] Fiala KA, Casa DJ, Roti MW. Rehydration with a caffeinated beverage during the nonexercise periods of 3 consecutive days of 2-a-day practices. Int J Sport Nutr Exerc Metab 2004;14(4):419–29.
[26] Armstrong LE, Pumerantz AC, Roti MW, et al. Fluid, electrolyte, and renal indices of hydration during 11 days of controlled caffeine consumption. Int J Sport Nutr Exerc Metab 2005;15(3):252–65.
[27] Roti MW, Casa DJ, Pumerantz AC, et al. Thermoregulatory responses to exercise in the heat: chronic caffeine intake has no effect. Aviat Space Environ Med 2006;77(2): 124–9.
[28] Almond CS, Shin AY, Fortescue EB, et al. Hyponatremia among runners in the Boston Marathon. N Engl J Med 2005;352(15):1550–6.
[29] Armstrong LE. Exertional hyponatremia. In: Armstrong LE, editor. Exertional heat illnesses. Champaign (IL): Human Kinetics; 2003. p. 103–35.
[30] Vrijens DM, Rehrer NJ. Sodium-free fluid ingestion decreases plasma sodium during exercise in the heat. J Appl Physiol 1999;86(6):1847–51.
[31] Speedy DB, Noakes TD, Kimber NE, et al. Fluid balance during and after an ironman triathlon. Clin J Sport Med 2001;11(1):44–50.
[32] Speedy DB, Noakes TD, Rogers IR, et al. Hyponatremia in ultradistance triathletes. Med Sci Sports Exerc 1999;31(6):809–15.
[33] Armstrong LE. Exertional hyponatraemia. J Sports Sci 2004;22(1):144–5.
[34] Twerenbold R, Knechtle B, Kakebeeke TH, et al. Effects of different sodium concentrations in replacement fluids during prolonged exercise in women. Br J Sports Med 2003;37(4): 300–3.
[35] Hew-Butler T, Almond C, Ayus JC, et al. Consensus statement of the 1st international exercise-associated hyponatremia consensus development conference, Cape Town, South Africa 2005. Clin J Sport Med 2005;15(4):208–13.
[36] Weschler LB. Exercise-associated hyponatraemia: a mathematical review. Sports Med 2005;35(10):899–922.
[37] Hew-Butler TD, Sharwood K, Collins M, et al. Sodium supplementation is not required to maintain serum sodium concentrations during an ironman triathlon. Br J Sports Med 2006;40(3):255–9.
[38] Montain SJ, Sawka MN, Wenger CB. Hyponatremia associated with exercise: risk factors and pathogenesis. Exerc Sport Sci Rev 2001;29(3):113–7.
[39] Convertino VA, Armstrong LE, Coyle EF, et al. American College of Sports Medicine position stand: exercise and fluid replacement. Med Sci Sports Exerc 1996;28(1): i–vii.
[40] Montain SJ, Cheuvront SN, Sawka MN. Exercise associated hyponatraemia: quantitative analysis to understand the aetiology. Br J Sports Med 2006;40(2):98–105.
[41] Baker LB, Munce TA, Kenney WL. Sex differences in voluntary fluid intake by older adults during exercise. Med Sci Sports Exerc 2005;37(5):789–96.
[42] Barr SI, Costill DL, Fink WJ. Fluid replacement during prolonged exercise: effects of water, saline, or no fluid. Med Sci Sports Exerc 1991;23(7):811–7.
[43] Speedy DB, Thompson JM, Rodgers I, et al. Oral salt supplementation during ultradistance exercise. Clin J Sport Med 2002;12(5):279–84.
[44] Weschler LB, Rehrer NJ. What can be concluded regarding water versus sports drinks from the Vrijens-Reher experiments? J Appl Physiol 2006;100(4):1433–4.
[45] Powers ME, Arnold BL, Weltman AL, et al. Creatine supplementation increases total body water without altering fluid distribution. J Athl Train 2003;38(1):44–50.
[46] Kilduff LP, Georgiades E, James N, et al. The effects of creatine supplementation on cardiovascular, metabolic, and thermoregulatory responses during exercise in the heat in endurance-trained humans. Int J Sport Nutr Exerc Metab 2004;14(4):443–60.
[47] Bailes JE, Cantu RC, Day AL. The neurosurgeon in sport: awareness of the risks of heatstroke and dietary supplements. Neurosurgery 2002;51(2):283–8.

[48] Terjung RL, Clarkson P, Eichner ER, et al. American College of Sports Medicine roundtable: the physiological and health effects of oral creatine supplementation. Med Sci Sports Exerc 2000;32(3):706–17.
[49] Demant TW, Rhodes EC. Effects of creatine supplementation on exercise performance. Sports Med 1999;28(1):49–60.
[50] Kern M, Podewils LJ, Vukovich M, et al. Physiological response to exercise in the heat following creatine supplementation. J Exerc Physiol 2001;4:18–27.
[51] Watson G, Casa D, Fiala KA, et al. Creatine use and exercise heat tolerance in dehydrated men. J Athl Train 2006;41(1):18–29.
[52] Weiss CA, Powers ME, Horodyski MB. Creatine supplementation does not alter the physiological response to exercise in the heat. J Athl Train 2003;38(2):S29.
[53] Schwellnus MP, Derman EW, Noakes TD. Aetiology of skeletal muscle 'cramps' during exercise: a novel hypothesis. J Sports Sci 1997;15(3):277–85.
[54] McGee SR. Muscle cramps. Arch Intern Med 1990;150(3):511–8.
[55] American Medical Association. International classification of diseases: manual of the international statistical classification of diseases, injuries, and causes of death, 9th revision. Chicago: AMA; 1998.
[56] Bergeron MF. Heat cramps during tennis: a case report. Int J Sport Nutr 1996;6(1):62–8.
[57] Stofan JR, Zachwieja JJ, Horswill CA, et al. Sweat and sodium losses in NCAA football players: a precursor to heat cramps? Int J Sport Nutr Exerc Metab 2005;15(6):641–52.
[58] Talbot JH. Heat cramps. Medicine. Baltimore: Williams and Wilkins; 1935. p. 323–76.
[59] Hubbard RW, Armstrong LE. The heat illnesses: biochemical, ultrastructural, and fluid-electrolyte considerations. In: Pandolf KB, Sawka MN, Gonzalez RR, editors. Human performance physiology and environmental medicine at terrestrial extremes. Traverse City: Cooper Publishing Group; 1988. p. 305–59.
[60] Armstrong LE. Considerations for replacement beverages: fluid-electrolyte balance and heat illness. In: Fluid replacement and heat stress. Washington, DC: National Academy Press; 1993. p. 37–54.
[61] Ladell WSS. Heat cramps. Lancet 1949;2:836–9.
[62] Bergeron MF. Exertional heat cramps. In: Armstrong LE, editor. Exertional heat illnesses. Champaign (IL): Human Kinetics; 2003. p. 91–102.
[63] Bergeron MF. Heat cramps: fluid and electrolyte challenges during tennis in the heat. J Sci Med Sport 2003;6(1):19–27.
[64] Coyle EF. Fluid and fuel intake during exercise. J Sports Sci 2004;22(1):39–55.
[65] Casa D. Proper hydration for distance running—identifying individual fluid needs. Track Coach 2004;167:5321–8.
[66] Armstrong LE, Hubbard RW, Szlyk PC, et al. Voluntary dehydration and electrolyte losses during prolonged exercise in the heat. Aviat Space Environ Med 1985;56(8):765–70.
[67] Rehrer NJ. Fluid and electrolyte balance in ultra-endurance sport. Sports Med 2001;31(10):701–15.
[68] Riedesel ML, Allen DY, Peake GT, et al. Hyperhydration with glycerol solutions. J Appl Physiol 1987;63(6):2262–8.
[69] Wingo JE, Casa DJ, Berger EM, et al. Influence of a pre-exercise glycerol hydration beverage on performance and physiologic function during mountain-bike races in the heat. J Athl Train 2004;39(2):169–75.
[70] Kavouras SA, Armstrong LE, Maresh CM, et al. Rehydration with glycerol: endocrine, cardiovascular, and thermoregulatory responses during exercise in the heat. J Appl Physiol 2006;100(2):442–50.
[71] Castellani JW, Maresh CM, Armstrong LE, et al. Intravenous vs. oral rehydration: effects on subsequent exercise-heat stress. J Appl Physiol 1997;82(3):799–806.
[72] Casa DJ, Maresh CM, Armstrong LE, et al. Intravenous versus oral rehydration during a brief period: responses to subsequent exercise in the heat. Med Sci Sports Exerc 2000;32(1):124–33.

[73] Figaro MK, Mack GW. Regulation of fluid intake in dehydrated humans: role of oropharyngeal stimulation. Am J Physiol 1997;272(6 Pt 2):R1740–6.
[74] Murray BM. Training the gut for competition. Curr Sports Med Rep 2006;5:161–4.
[75] Casa DJ, Clarkson PM, Roberts WO. American College of Sports Medicine roundtable on hydration and physical activity: consensus statements. Curr Sports Med Rep 2005;4(3):115–27.

Clin Sports Med 26 (2007) 17–36
CLINICS IN SPORTS MEDICINE

ELSEVIER
SAUNDERS

Protein Requirements and Recommendations for Athletes: Relevance of Ivory Tower Arguments for Practical Recommendations

Kevin D. Tipton, PhD*, Oliver C. Witard, MSc
School of Sport and Exercise Sciences, University of Birmingham, Edgbaston, Birmingham B29 5SA, United Kingdom

Protein nutrition for athletes has long been a topic of interest. From the legendary Greek wrestler Milo–purported to eat copious amounts of beef during his five successive Olympic titles–to modern athletes consuming huge amounts of supplements, protein intake has been considered paramount. Recommendations for protein intake for athletes has not been without controversy, however. In general, scientific opinion on this controversy seems to divide itself into two camps–those who believe participation in exercise and sport increases the nutritional requirement for protein and those who believe protein requirements for athletes and exercising individuals are no different from the requirements for sedentary individuals. There seems to be evidence for both arguments. Although this issue may be scientifically relevant, from a practical perspective, the requirement for protein–as most often defined–may not be applicable to most athletes.

The argument over protein requirements for athletes and active individuals often takes a general form; requirements for athletes are compared with the requirements set for sedentary individuals. Often, the athletic population participates in either endurance exercise or resistance exercise. Even this division does not take into account, however, the myriad physiologic and metabolic demands of training that inevitably vary for athletes involved in different sports. The demands of training may vary within a particular sport or in individuals. In this article, the authors argue that the controversy over protein requirements that is expressed often in the literature–although interesting from a scientific standpoint–is irrelevant for athletes, coaches, and nutrition practitioners.

Contributing to the controversy is the perception of the definition of protein requirement. Athletes define their dietary requirement for protein differently than scientists. Typically, the definition for the requirement of protein is based on nitrogen balance (ie, the minimum amount of protein necessary to balance

*Corresponding author. *E-mail address*: k.d.tipton@bham.ac.uk (K.D. Tipton).

0278-5919/07/$ – see front matter
doi:10.1016/j.csm.2006.11.003
© 2007 Elsevier Inc. All rights reserved.
sportsmed.theclinics.com

all nitrogen losses and maintain nitrogen balance). This approach, or something similar, has been used to determine the estimates of protein intake necessary for athletes [1–4]. More complex models of protein requirements include consideration for the metabolic demands of the body [5]. The obligatory and adaptive demands for amino nitrogen are included in this model. Although these models have been used to set requirements for sedentary populations and to estimate requirements for athletes, it is unlikely that athletes consider them to be the appropriate measuring stick to make recommendations of protein intake that would be of maximum benefit.

This article addresses the issue of protein intake for athletes from a practical standpoint. The background information from previous studies has been presented in many excellent reviews that have examined the issue extensively [6–18], so this information is presented only briefly here. The focus instead is on how–in the authors' view–various factors involved in protein nutrition may influence the adaptations that result from training and nutritional intake, and how this information may be used by practitioners, coaches, and athletes to determine appropriate protein intakes during training for optimal competitive results.

CONTROVERSY

The argument has been made that regular exercise, particularly in elite athletes with highly demanding training regimens, increases protein requirements over those for sedentary individuals. This argument is often based on nitrogen balance. Several well-controlled studies have shown that nitrogen balance in athletes is greater than in inactive controls [1,3,4,19]. Increased protein needs may come from increased amino acid oxidation during exercise [20–23] or growth and repair of muscle tissue. Muscle protein synthesis (MPS) is increased after resistance [24–26] and endurance exercise [27,28], suggesting that additional protein would be necessary to provide amino acids for the increased protein synthesis. Increased synthesis is ostensibly necessary for production of new myofibrillar proteins for muscle growth during resistance training and for mitochondrial biogenesis during endurance training.

In contrast, it has been extensively argued that exercise, even extensive, prolonged, and intense exercise, does not increase the dietary requirement for protein [9,14,15,18,29–32]. The argument is often based on the fact that exercise has been shown to increase the efficiency of use of amino acids from ingested protein. Butterfield and others [29,30,33] demonstrated this concept in a series of classic experiments showing that even at relatively low protein intakes and negative energy balance, nitrogen balance was improved when exercise was performed. More recently, it has been shown that exercise training increases muscle protein balance [26,34], suggesting that the reuse of amino acids from muscle protein breakdown is more efficient. This notion was investigated in a prospective, longitudinal study on the whole-body protein level using stable isotopic tracers [35]. Whole-body protein balance was reduced in novice weightlifters after training, suggesting that protein requirements would be less with regular exercise training.

A common criticism of the studies that show increased use of amino acids with exercise is that the intensity or duration of exercise is not as great as that practiced by top sport athletes, and the requirements would be underestimated [16–18]. Many studies have shown that amino acid oxidation is elevated during exercise [22,23,36,37]. Animal studies have shown that exercise of sufficient intensity and duration may result in a catabolic state after exercise. MPS is decreased after exercise at high intensities and long duration [38,39]. It also has been reported that low-intensity endurance and resistance exercise does not stimulate MPS [40,41]. These results, together with the data indicating that higher intensity exercise increases MPS [24–26], suggest that there may be a continuum of exercise intensity in which the response of muscle protein metabolism changes (Fig. 1). At lower intensities, there is no response, but as intensity increases, MPS is stimulated. At the highest levels of exercise intensity and duration, however, the impact of the exercise reduces the response of MPS. Protein requirements may be related to the intensity and duration of the exercise that is practiced.

Arguments against protein requirements often are based on difficulties showing increased muscle mass at higher levels of protein intake. At best, studies are equivocal. Although studies have shown gains in muscle mass at higher protein intakes [42,43], a meta-analysis concluded that protein supplements had no impact on lean body mass during training [44]. When the apparent increases in nitrogen balance are extrapolated to gains in lean body mass, the calculations suggest gains that are physiologically impossible–on the order of 200 to 500 g/d [1,3,4]. These results show the tendency for nitrogen balance methods to overestimate nitrogen balance at high intakes, perhaps owing to increases in the urea pool size [13]. Suffice to say that there are studies providing evidence

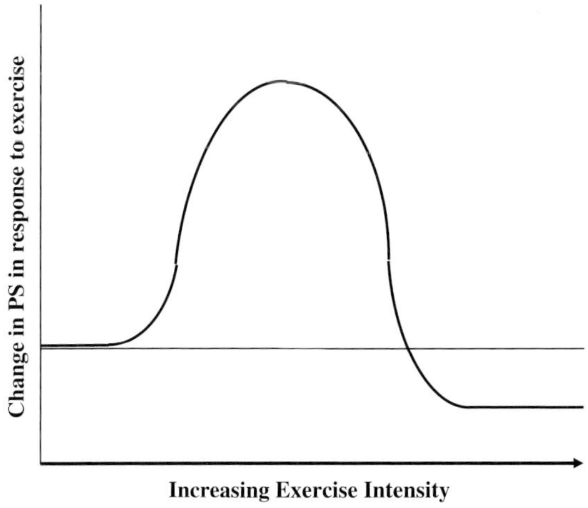

Fig. 1. Proposed response of muscle protein synthesis (PS) after exercise as exercise intensity increases.

for increased protein requirements for athletes and the opposite. These arguments are described in detail in other articles [11–13,15,16,18].

METHODOLOGIC CONSIDERATIONS

Methodologic inadequacies remain partly responsible for current difficulties in assessing protein requirements of the human diet for exercise. In terms of experimental design, most studies involve measurements of nitrogen losses or tracer-labeled amino acid oxidation rates [45].

Nitrogen balance techniques are used most often to estimate protein requirements by quantification of all protein that is consumed and all nitrogen that is excreted. Positive nitrogen balance indicates an anabolic situation, and negative balance indicates protein catabolism. Healthy adults who are not growing should be in nitrogen balance over a given period of time; however, for a short period, balance may be positive or negative. Nitrogen balance is indirectly reflective of a complex series of ongoing metabolic changes in (1) whole-body protein turnover, (2) amino acid oxidation, (3) urea production, and (4) nitrogen excretion during fasting, fed, postprandial, and postabsorptive periods of the day [46].

Nitrogen balance data are not without inherent problems. Limitations of nitrogen balance have been well covered previously [10,46–50]. Suffice to say that criticisms of nitrogen balance are multiple and include a lack of sensitivity because it involves only gross measures of nitrogen intake and excretion [47]; difficulties in precisely quantifying nitrogen losses, which may be particularly important for active individuals [51]; changes in size of the body urea pool [10]; mismatches between nitrogen balance and measurable changes in protein mass [11,16], especially at high intakes [11]; poor reproducibility [49]; and accommodation by limitation of other processes at nitrogen balance with low protein intakes [50].

Application of nitrogen balance measurements to athletes may be especially unsuitable. For a strength athlete, whose goal is to increase lean body mass and ultimately muscle strength and size, protein requirements set to attain nitrogen balance are inappropriate; rather, the athlete aims to consume enough dietary protein to induce a positive nitrogen balance [11]. It may be more appropriate to discuss protein requirements with respect to the strength athlete as the effect of dietary protein on protein synthesis and breakdown [51]. Similarly, consideration of nitrogen balance only may not be appropriate for an endurance athlete; balance may be attained, but with a compromise in some physiologically relevant processes, such as upregulation of enzyme activity, capillarization, or mitochondrial biogenesis after endurance training [16]. The nitrogen balance approach underlies the establishment of dietary reference intake for protein in sedentary individuals, so comparison of like with like makes feasible the argument that nitrogen balance should be used for determination of protein requirements for athletic populations.

Other methods for determining protein requirements include use of stable isotopic tracers and functional indicators of protein adequacy [10]. Use of these methods has been the source of a great deal of controversy over the years for athletic and nonathletic populations [10,16,18,45,49,52].

PROTEIN AND PERFORMANCE

Although nitrogen balance and stable isotope studies are of great interest in building an experimental database to support, refute, or challenge official published levels of requirements, from a practical standpoint, coaches, athletes, and individuals involved in daily exercise regimens are not usually interested in the scientific debate over the issue of protein requirements. Performance is ultimately the only outcome that is important for athletes. Many authors have made this point, yet the studies that have attempted to investigate the influence of protein intake on performance have been scarce [10,11,16,18,51]. Millward [10] stated, "Thus, the key test of adequacy of either protein or amino acid intake must be the long-term response in terms of the specific function of interest." This key test would vary for each type of exercise training performed, each sport, each position within a particular sport, and even among individuals participating in any given event or sharing a position (eg, an American football quarterback compared with a running back). Energy balance, intake of other nutrients, and individual genetic makeup all contribute to the response to training and nutrient intake, and the influence of the amount of protein ingested per day on performance for an athlete varies and often is difficult to determine.

There are ample limitations for determination of optimal protein intake by measurement of performance. These limitations have been articulated previously [11,13,16,18,51] and include difficulty, if not impossibility, in controlling innumerable physiologic variables (eg, training status, training details, energy balance, and standardization of life aspects such as sleep, work, and emotional upheavals) and inherent difficulty in defining the appropriate end points to be measured and the insensitivity of performance and end point measures [11,16,18,51].

Determination of appropriate protein intake to optimize performance, by any method, is limited by the definition of the population to be targeted. Generally, studies broadly divide athletes into strength or power athletes and endurance athletes. These broad distinctions may not be specific enough to provide appropriate protein intake information for many athletes. There have been attempts to categorize various athletic groups further. Tarnopolsky [16] considered that endurance athletes may be divided into three broad categories and estimated protein needs for these groups. Delineations such as these provide more information for practitioners, but as is pointed out in Tarnopolsky's article, there are individuals who do not fit the broad categorizations. It seems clear that, at this juncture, there are ample gaps in knowledge that do not allow general recommendations that may be meaningful to all athletes. Football and rugby players incorporate a great deal of power and endurance training. A decathlete, by definition, participates in quite varied training. Gender is an important factor to consider [16,23,53], but few data exist on performance measures on different protein intakes for men and women. To recommend a specific number of grams of protein to all participants in a broad category of athletes seems nonsensical. Protein recommendations are best made based on the individual circumstances of each athlete.

HABITUAL INTAKES OF PROTEIN FOR ATHLETES

Within the limitations available, determination of protein requirements in studies to date often suggests that protein intake should be greater for athletes than for sedentary individuals. Generally, the range given is 1.2 to about 2.0 g protein/kg body weight per day [1,11,12,16,23,53,54]. As mentioned, many authors dispute these higher estimates and maintain that exercise does not increase requirements, even among highly trained athletes expending large amounts of energy [13–15,31,45,55]. An often noted point is that even if the highest of estimates are the true requirement, it is likely that for most athletes, the point is moot. More recently published articles have provided summaries of protein intake for endurance [16] and strength-based [11] athletes. It is clear from these studies that reported dietary protein intakes are normally greater than even the increased estimates proposed. Such athletes are at little risk of protein deficiency, provided that a net energy balance is achieved to maintain body weight, and sound nutritional practices are adhered to. Supplemental protein seems to be unnecessary for most athletes who consume a varied diet that contains complete protein foods and meets energy needs.

As Tarnopolsky [16] pointed out, however, the range of protein intakes indicates that there are numerous individuals, perhaps 20%, who may consume levels of protein below some estimates of requirements for sedentary individuals. Perhaps individuals at greatest risk of consuming insufficient protein are those whose lifestyle combines other factors known to increase protein needs with intense training and competition, including individuals with insufficient energy intake, vegetarians, athletes competing in weight-class competitions, athletes participating in a suddenly increased level of training (eg, training camps), and individuals undergoing weight-loss programs. Generally, the evidence available indicates that most athletes who could be considered at risk tend to eat ample protein. The ranges indicate, however, that certain individuals may be at risk of insufficient protein intake, assuming that protein requirements fall in the elevated ranges.

Coaches, trainers, and athletes are apt to question whether a vegetarian diet can provide adequate protein to meet the increased dietary needs of highly trained athletes [56]. Concerns may stem from the ability of a vegetarian diet to provide all essential amino acids (EAA) in the diet. Because a vegetarian diet is a plant-based diet, the quality of the ingested protein may be questioned. All EAA and nonessential amino acids can be supplied by plant food sources alone, provided that a variety of foods are consumed, and energy intake remains adequate to meet these needs [56]. Of particular concern, however, are individuals who avoid all animal protein sources (ie, vegans) because plant proteins may be limited in amino acids containing lysine, threonine, tryptophan, or sulfur [57]. If the diet is too restricted, suboptimal mineral and protein intake is possible.

Although most vegetarian diets meet or exceed dietary recommendations for protein, they often provide less protein than do nonvegetarian diets [58]. Vegetarian athletes are likely to consume protein of lower quality that may increase the amount of protein required to meet needs [12,13,59]. Perhaps more importantly, use of ingested amino acids, particularly by muscle [12,60–62], and nitrogen balance [63–65] may be less with plant protein sources. These concerns suggest that it is possible that some vegetarian athletes may need to consider carefully the amount of protein intake necessary to accomplish the same training and competitive goals. In studies to date, well-planned, appropriately supplemented vegetarian diets seem to support effectively parameters that would affect athletic performance [57], albeit data on athletic populations are scarce. Similar increases in muscle strength and cross-sectional area in older men eating primarily meat protein or soy protein were noted during 12 weeks of resistance exercise training [66], suggesting that dependence on predominantly plant protein sources does not influence the response to training when dietary energy and protein intakes are matched. The issue of protein quality is recognized as a potential concern for individuals who avoid all animal protein sources (ie, vegans); however it is unlikely that concerns would apply to every vegan athlete.

INFLUENCE OF ENERGY INTAKE ON PROTEIN USE

In any discussion of protein requirements and recommendations, the influence of energy intake must be considered. Energy intake is likely to have as much influence on protein requirements as does protein intake itself [67]. It is impossible to maintain positive nitrogen balance in the face of energy deficits; even given high protein intakes [30,33,67]. It has been estimated that approximately one third of the variation in nitrogen balance among individuals may be accounted for by energy intake [68]. Early work showed that athletes gain strength and maintain muscle mass even during periods of low protein intake, provided that energy intake is sufficient [69]. During resistance exercise training, it has been shown that positive energy balance is more important than increased protein to elicit gains in lean body mass [70,71]. Energy intake must be carefully considered before making any recommendation for protein intake to a given individual.

The influence of energy balance on protein metabolism and balance suggests another area of potential concern for some athletes. Athletes who restrict energy intake may need to be especially conscious of protein intake. Athletes involved in weight-class sports (eg, boxing and wrestling), esthetic sports (eg, figure skating, gymnastics, and diving), and sports in which excess weight may be deemed to impair performance (eg, horse-racing [jockeys], rowing, or distance running) may need to be particularly vigilant. Even so, there is no reason to suspect that all or even many of these athletes need to ingest protein in excess of their current diet. It is often thought that a prominent example of a population that may need special attention is female, particularly young, gymnasts. It is possible that protein needs are greater because nutritional assessments of female gymnasts indicate that many have an energy intake lower than energy expenditure [72,73]. Female gymnasts have been shown to consume less protein than female controls, and this intake is related to lower whole-body protein balance [72]. If female gymnasts are examined in more detail, it seems that most of even this potentially vulnerable population of athletes consume enough protein. In Table 1, calculations are shown for the protein intake for a small, approximately 45-kg athlete and a possible range of energy and protein intakes. For all but the lowest energy and protein intakes, sufficient protein would be ingested. Although most gymnasts, similar to other athletes, likely habitually consume ample protein to support their training and competition, these data suggest that some individuals within this population may be in need of particular attention when recommending protein intakes. Other athletes with similar training and psychological issues also may be at risk.

Many athletes desire to decrease body mass with as small a reduction of lean mass as possible. Numerous studies support a role for high-protein diets in promoting greater body weight and fat loss while maintaining lean mass compared with diets low in protein composition [74–79]. These studies investigated weight loss in obese or overweight populations, so the applicability of these findings to athletes is questionable. Nevertheless, it is possible that increased dietary protein intake may have relevance to some athletes who desire loss of body mass with minimal reductions of lean mass and perhaps performance.

The leucine content of the diet has been hypothesized to be a potential mechanism important in maintaining lean mass and promoting fat loss [80]. Leucine is a key regulator of MPS [38,81–83], and maintenance of MPS during hypocaloric conditions may mediate maintenance of lean body mass. Support for this idea is found in a study by Harber and colleagues [84]. MPS was increased after a period of high protein intake compared with higher carbohydrate intake. Although this concept provides a rationale for use of higher protein intakes for athletes desiring to reduce body mass, it has never been tested in exercising individuals over a period of training and may not apply. Bolster and coworkers [85] showed that MPS was reduced after exercise in runners on a very high protein diet compared with more moderate protein intakes. Studies in exercising

Table 1
Estimated protein intake for a female gymnast consuming 20%, 15%, and 10% of energy intake as protein

Energy intake (MJ/d)	6.7	8.4
P/E[a]	g protein intake/kg body weight/d	
20	1.77	2.22
15	1.33	1.66
10	0.88	1.11

Energy intake values represent a range of possible intakes based on previous intake data [72] and estimates from Harris-Benedict equation.

[a]P/E ratio is defined as the percentage contribution of protein to total energy intake.

humans from Wolfe's laboratory (Elliot et al, unpublished data) and others [86] fail to show that extra leucine provides additional stimulation of MPS.

There are potential drawbacks of higher protein intakes during hypocaloric situations–and possibly during energy balance–that must be avoided if performance is not to suffer. Performance of well-trained cyclists was impaired on a diet in which protein intake was elevated in place of carbohydrates [87]. If carbohydrate intake is compromised to increase protein intake, glycogen stores may be reduced, and training intensity for some athletes (ie, athletes whose training involves high-intensity or prolonged workouts) could suffer. Another possible problem with ingestion of high-protein diets is the potential for instigating negative nitrogen balance if the high protein intake is curtailed. Quevedo and coworkers [88] showed that nitrogen balance was reduced for a time after a reduction in protein intake, but that nitrogen balance slowly returns to zero balance at the lower intakes. The likely explanation for this decrease in nitrogen balance after a reduction in protein intake lies in the pathways of protein and amino acid degradation. It is likely that degradative pathways are upregulated during times of high protein intake, and the decreased intake level is insufficient to replenish losses [10,88]. These studies were conducted at rest during energy balance. It is possible that this loss of nitrogen would be even greater in athletes during hypocaloric situations, even given the known upregulation of protein use owing to exercise [30]. The applicability of this model to well-trained athletes at high levels of exercise is unknown. Nevertheless, careful consideration of training and competitive demands for each athlete must precede recommendations for increased protein intakes.

FACTORS THAT AFFECT USE OF INGESTED PROTEIN

Estimates of protein requirements for athletes and all other populations are based on the concept that the adaptations owing to protein ingestion depend solely on the amount of protein ingested on a daily basis given the training demands for a given group (eg, endurance or resistance-trained athletes). The influence that other dietary factors, such as type of protein being consumed, and that other nutrients in the diet and timing of protein ingestion may have on the use of the ingested protein and the adaptations stemming from intake of the protein is not taken into account. In recent years, a growing body of evidence based on acute metabolic studies suggests that the metabolic response to protein and amino acid ingestion, particularly in muscle, is far more complex than is implied simply by consideration of the amount of protein ingested on a daily basis. For any given protein intake, the metabolic response–and presumably the adaptations in the muscle–would vary and depend on a variety of factors involved in the form and process of nutrient intake.

The composition of the ingested protein would influence the response to a given diet. The impact of protein quality on protein requirements has long been recognized as an important consideration for making nutritional recommendations. On a whole-body level, studies suggest that although vegetarian diets may be sufficient for positive nitrogen balance, reliance on animal proteins results in superior balance [63–65]. The purported superiority of animal proteins may not be as clear, however, as some studies indicate [59].

Whole-body studies may not give a clear picture of the importance of protein intake to other tissues, particularly muscle. In a series of experiments involving modeling based on stable isotopes, the complexities of use of amino acids from meals including different types of proteins has been examined. In general, use of amino acids from animal proteins (eg, milk) is greater than plant proteins (eg, wheat) [60–62], but differences exist even among different plant proteins [60–62,89,90]. These data suggest that amino acids from different protein sources may be preferentially used by different tissues. Amino acids ingested as milk proteins are taken up in greater amounts by peripheral (ie, muscle) rather than splanchnic tissues [61,90]. There is an interaction of protein type and the amount of protein ingested, such that use of amino acids from ingested animal proteins is diminished less than plant proteins at higher protein intake levels [62]. Although these investigations were performed in resting subjects, and the relevancy to athletes may be questioned, these data make it clear that use of amino acids from ingested proteins may be handled differently depending on the type of protein that is ingested. These results may be interpreted to support the idea that adaptations to diets with different types of proteins during training may be different even if similar amounts of proteins are ingested.

Data on amino acid use from various proteins after exercise are limited. Consistent with the data based on modeling in resting adults, Phillips and colleagues [12] reported that uptake of amino acids from milk proteins into muscle is greater than from soy protein after resistance exercise. In resting volunteers, casein may provide a superior anabolic response compared with whey proteins on a whole-body level [91]. On a muscle level after resistance exercise, however, the differences in amino acid uptake between casein and whey proteins are less clear [92].

Other nutrients ingested concurrently with protein also influence use of the ingested amino acids. At rest, whole-body amino acid retention is increased when proteins are consumed with carbohydrates [93,94]. Although the total retention of ingested amino acids is greater with carbohydrate than fat ingestion [93,94], the uptake into body regions seems to be differentially affected. Concurrent fat ingestion resulted in greater retention of ingested amino acids in peripheral tissues than did sucrose ingestion [93]. Consistent with these results in resting subjects, it has been shown that carbohydrate ingestion increases the use of amino acids ingested concomitantly after resistance exercise [95–98], an effect likely mediated by the insulin response [99]. Preliminary evidence suggests that lipid increases amino acid use of milk proteins ingested during recovery from resistance exercise [100]. The mechanism for this effect remains to be elucidated. The results from several studies examining use of ingested proteins after exercise are summarized in Fig. 2. Taken together, these results show that ingestion of a particular amount of protein stimulates metabolic processes that are influenced by the nutrients ingested concurrently. These acute responses suggest that adaptations in athletes could be independent of the amount of protein ingested.

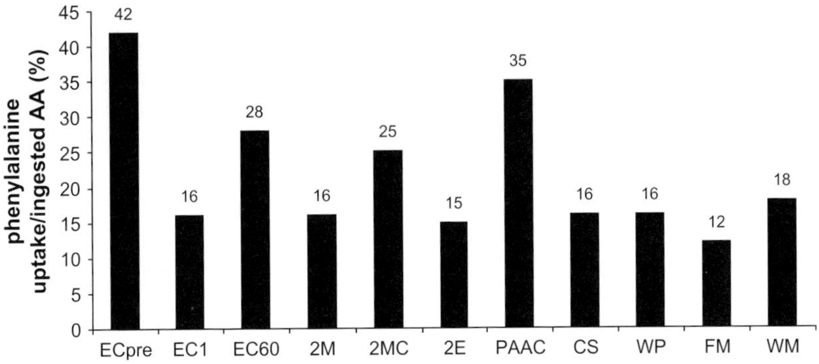

Fig. 2. Use of ingested amino acids for muscle protein accretion from various sources of amino acids ingested after resistance exercise. Use is represented by % phenylalanine taken up across the leg relative to ingested at various times after exercise. All uptake was calculated as area under the curve of net balance for 3 hours. ECpre = 6 g essential amino acids (EAA) + 35 g carbohydrate (CHO) ingested pre-exercise [103]; EC1 = 6 g EAA + 35 g CHO ingested <1 minute postexercise [103]; EC60 = 6 g EAA + 35 g CHO ingested 1 hour postexercise [114]; 2M = 6 g mixed amino acids (MAA) ingested 1 hour and 2 hours postexercise [98]; 2MC = 6 g MAA + 35 g CHO ingested 1 hour and 2 hours postexercise [98]; 2E = 6 g EAA ingested 1 hour and 2 hours postexercise [95]; PAAC = amino acid (4.9 g AA), protein (17.5 g whey protein) and CHO (77.4 g) mixture ingested 1 hour postexercise [97]; CS = 20 g casein protein ingested 1 hour postexercise [92]; WP = 20 g whey protein ingested 1 hour postexercise [92]; FM = 237 g of fat-free milk ingested 1 hour postexercise [100]; WM = 237 g of whole milk ingested 1 hour postexercise [100]. Use of the ingested amino acids varies depending on the type of amino acids, timing of ingestion, and coingestion of other nutrients.

In addition to other nutrients and the type of protein, the metabolic response of muscle may be affected by the timing of the ingestion of amino acids or protein in relation to the exercise bout. Timing of ingestion of a mixture of carbohydrate, fat, and protein [101]; carbohydrates alone [102]; and EAA plus carbohydrates [103] would influence the anabolic response to resistance exercise. It seems that different sources of amino acids do not engender the same response to varied timing of ingestion. In a previous study, the anabolic response to ingestion of a solution of EAA and carbohydrates immediately before exercise was approximately three times that of the response when the solution was ingested after exercise [103]. In a more recent study using an identical protocol, however, the response to ingestion of whey proteins immediately before exercise was similar to that after exercise [104]. It seems that not only timing of ingestion, but also the interaction of the type of protein with the timing determines the anabolic response in muscle.

Taken together, the anabolic response of muscle depends not only on the form of the ingested amino acids, but also on the nutrients ingested in association with the amino acids and the timing of the ingestion in relation to exercise–not to mention the interaction of all these factors. The complexity involved in assessing the relationship of the anabolic response to exercise and nutrition is readily apparent. Consideration of only the amount of protein ingested on a daily basis does not provide a complete picture of the metabolic situation that would influence the adaptations to training and nutrition. Broad recommendations for a particular amount of protein for all athletes or even subgroups of those involved in various types of sport without consideration of many other factors seems nonsensical.

IMPLICATIONS OF SHORT-TERM STUDIES FOR LONG-TERM ADAPTATIONS

The conclusion that use of amino acids from ingested protein varies depending on the factors discussed previously is based on studies that acutely measure changes in net muscle protein balance (NBAL). These investigations often make use of stable isotopic tracers, arteriovenous balance, or muscle biopsy samples to examine the changes in muscle metabolism resulting from an intervention. The assumption is made that changes in metabolism observed during short-term measurement periods represent the potential for long-term changes that may affect adaptations to protein ingestion.

In Wolfe's laboratory in Galveston, Texas, the potential for acute studies to represent long-term changes has been investigated. Results from these studies are consistent with the notion that determinations of protein use based on results from acute studies are representative of those that may occur over longer periods of training. Stable isotopic tracers were used to measure MPS and NBAL in volunteers over a 24-hour period under two conditions: (1) while resting and (2) during a 24-hour period when they performed resistance exercise and ingested EAA [105]. Comparison of the results during a 3-hour period after exercise (ie, comparable to the time typically used in acute studies) were made with results obtained over 24 hours. Exercise plus EAA ingestion increased the rate of MPS measured over 24 hours and improved NBAL compared with rest. The difference between rest and exercise plus amino acid ingestion was similar whether determined over 3 hours or a full 24-hour period, suggesting that acute changes in NBAL represent those that occur over longer periods.

If the acute response of muscle to exercise and nutrient intake is to be deemed representative of long-term changes, the response of NBAL before and after resistance exercise training must be constant. In other words, changes in the acute response over a period of training and dietary manipulation would mean that measurement of the acute response before training could not be extrapolated to estimate the entire response to training. In a recent study, we determined the acute response of NBAL to resistance exercise during ingestion of EAA in untrained volunteers before and after a period of resistance training (Tipton et al., unpublished results). The response of NBAL to resistance exercise and EAA was similar before and after 16 weeks of training consistent with the notion that extrapolation of results from the acute study could be used to determine the use of amino acids from protein ingestion over longer periods. Similarly, Phillips and colleagues [12] reported that the anabolic response of muscle NBAL to ingestion of milk and soy protein after exercise successfully predicted the accumulation of muscle mass in healthy young volunteers over a 12-week period. Another study in which NBAL was measured before and after 28 days of bed rest with and without EAA supplementation [106] offers further support for the efficacy of short-term studies. Positive NBAL resulted from ingestion of EAA before and after bed rest, although the response was attenuated after the extended inactivity. Comparison of muscle mass lost during bed rest from dual-energy x-ray absorptiometry measures with estimates based on extrapolation from the acute NBAL measurement was quite similar [106].

Finally, molecular data indicate that an acute bout of exercise impacts gene expression [107], primarily through the transcriptional and translational signaling pathways [108,109]. The ability of researchers to examine the molecular mechanisms behind training-induced changes has increased in recent years [107]. These types of studies have provided information suggesting that many long-term training–induced adaptations are the result of the cumulative effect of the acute, transient changes that occur during recovery from each individual exercise bout [110]. It seems that the type of nutrients consumed after exercise affects the regulation of metabolic gene expression and the adaptations to training [111]. The transient nature of the response to exercise and feeding on the metabolic [18,112] and molecular levels [108,110,113] is consistent with the notion that adaptation to exercise training depends on the accumulation of the responses to each individual exercise bout [108–111,113]. All of these results support the use of acute studies for determination of the impact of various nutritional and exercise regimens on protein use and providing information on the potential for long-term adaptations.

SUMMARY AND RECOMMENDATIONS

The debate concerning protein requirements is interesting from a scientific standpoint, but is likely to be ignored by athletes in favor of articulating protein recommendations for each athlete. Most athletes seem to ingest sufficient protein. Some individual athletes, particularly within certain populations (vegetarians, athletes involved in weight-class sports, female endurance runners, and individuals involved in weight-loss regimens), are potentially at risk of not consuming sufficient high-quality protein, however, and perhaps extra attention may be warranted for these types of athletes. Broad, generalized recommendations do not seem to offer much use other than as an overall guide. Many factors must be considered for each individual athlete before a recommended protein intake should be determined. It is possible that some athletes may need to consider increasing protein intakes, especially if energy balance is an issue. If protein is increased at the expense of carbohydrates, however, the performance of some athletes may suffer. If glycogen status is not imperative for training demands, higher amounts of protein may be well tolerated. Careful consideration of the competitive goals and training demands should be an important aspect of any nutritional recommendation.

Protein intake is fundamental aspect of an athlete's diet. There can be little doubt that higher protein intakes would not be a problem for many athletes, and there are situations where it may be warranted. Careful examination of the energetic and metabolic demands of the training is crucial for determination of optimal protein intake. A "first, do no harm" approach is likely to be the optimal strategy. As such, risk/benefit analysis would be prudent. There seems to be little health risk of higher protein intakes until very high levels. Many believe that there is no risk until intakes reach approximately 40% of energy intakes, and it would be unusual for athletes to ingest protein at that level. A male athlete consuming 3000 kcal/d would have to eat 300 g of protein (ie, 3.75 g/kg/d for an 80-kg athlete) to reach these levels. There is no evidence that ingestion of protein at that level is beneficial, but the likelihood of a health risk is slight.

Increasing habitual protein intake is unnecessary and provides little benefit for most athletes who consume a well-balanced diet that meets energy demands and includes varied sources of high-quality protein. There are situations in which a particular athlete may benefit from higher protein intakes. Increasingly, studies suggest that increasing protein may be beneficial for some, perhaps especially so for individuals in weight-loss situations. Much more work needs to be done in this area. There also are athletes for whom high protein intakes may be unnecessary, but do have possible utility that has yet to be determined. If it is determined that protein intake at these levels is not detrimental for optimal training and competition, there may be no reason to limit protein intake.

Finally, it seems that a simple approach to determining appropriate intake may be best. Determination of the optimal energy intake to balance training demands is crucial. Careful consideration of ample carbohydrate intake should be a priority, particularly for athletes engaged in repeated, high-intensity training sessions. Protein intake can be set at a level that is not harmful and may be beneficial. Fat intake should not be so low that deficiencies of essential fatty acids are an issue. Fat intake is associated with a more enjoyable diet, and so overly restricting fats may lead to compliance issues. There is no reason to incorporate dietary regimens that would not be followed.

In the authors' view, much of the protein requirement controversy is really much ado about nothing. It is an interesting, ivory-tower debate that has yet to be resolved. From a practical standpoint, however, habitual protein intakes are fine for most athletes. There are individual athletes for whom increased protein intake may be warranted so long as the coach, physician, and nutritionist have carefully weighed the risks and benefits. There is no reason to recommend protein supplements per se because there is no evidence that supplements work better than foods. The amount of protein necessary to increase muscle mass by 5 kg for an 80-kg male athlete is estimated in Table 2. Even considering the broad assumptions made, it is clear from these calculations that very little additional protein is necessary to support gains in muscle mass, and that it is not difficult to obtain any extra protein from foods.

Table 2
Example of protein intake necessary to increase muscle protein by 5 kg over 1 year in an 80-kg male athlete

All calculations assume
Muscle content = 75% water and 25% protein
Only 1.25 kg of 5 kg increase in LBM is derived from protein
Calculation 1—Required protein intake (assuming all ingested protein enters the muscle)
1.25 kg protein = 1250 g
1250 g/80 kg/365 d = 0.04 g/kg/BM/d
0.04 g/kg/d × 80 kg = 3.2 g protein/d
3.6 g protein = ~100 mL skim milk
Calculation 2—Required protein intake (assuming 25% of ingested protein enters the muscle)
0.04 g/kg/d × 4 = 0.16 g/kg/d
0.16 g/kg/d × 80 kg = 12.8 g protein/d
14.4 g protein = ~400 mL skim milk

Abbreviations: BM; body mass; LBM; lean body mass.

For athletes who are best served staying at energy balance, consuming a well-balanced diet that includes sufficient carbohydrates to fuel training and ensure performance and protein from a variety of sources should be key. For athletes interested in gaining muscle mass, an increase in energy intake, including a relatively high proportion of protein, is likely to be the primary objective. For athletes interested in losing mass and experiencing negative energy balance, a relatively high protein intake may be warranted within the context of preserving intake of other essential nutrients. Particular care must be taken to ensure sufficient carbohydrate intake as well.

References

[1] Lemon PW, Tarnopolsky MA, MacDougall JD, et al. Protein requirements and muscle mass/strength changes during intensive training in novice bodybuilders. J Appl Physiol 1992;73:767–75.
[2] Lemon PW, Dolny DG, Yarasheski KE. Moderate physical activity can increase dietary protein needs. Can J Appl Physiol 1997;22:494–503.
[3] Tarnopolsky MA, MacDougall JD, Atkinson SA. Influence of protein intake and training status on nitrogen balance and lean body mass. J Appl Physiol 1988;64:187–93.
[4] Tarnopolsky MA, Atkinson SA, MacDougall JD, et al. Evaluation of protein requirements for trained strength athletes. J Appl Physiol 1992;73:1986–95.
[5] Millward DJ. An adaptive metabolic demand model for protein and amino acid requirements. Br J Nutr 2003;90:249–60.
[6] Lemon PW. Do athletes need more dietary protein and amino acids? Int J Sport Nutr 1995;5(Suppl):S39–61.
[7] Lemon PW. Is increased dietary protein necessary or beneficial for individuals with a physically active lifestyle? Nutr Rev 1996;54:S169–75.
[8] Lemon PW. Beyond the zone: protein needs of active individuals. J Am Coll Nutr 2000;19:513S–21S.
[9] Millward DJ, Bowtell JL, Pacy P, et al. Physical activity, protein metabolism and protein requirements. Proc Nutr Soc 1994;53:223–40.

[10] Millward DJ. Inherent difficulties in defining amino acid requirements. In: Committee on Military Nutrition Research, editor. The role of protein and amino acids in sustaining and enhancing performance. Washington, DC: National Academy Press; 1999. p. 169–216.
[11] Phillips SM. Protein requirements and supplementation in strength sports. Nutrition 2004;20:689–95.
[12] Phillips SM, Hartman JW, Wilkinson SB. Dietary protein to support anabolism with resistance exercise in young men. J Am Coll Nutr 2005;24:134S–9S.
[13] Phillips SM. Dietary protein for athletes: from requirements to metabolic advantage. Appl Physiol Nutr Metab 2006, in press.
[14] Rennie MJ. Physical exertion, amino acid and protein metabolism, and protein requirements. In: Committee on Military Nutrition Research, editor. The role of protein and amino acids in sustaining and enhancing performance. Washington, DC: National Academy Press; 1999. p. 243–53.
[15] Rennie MJ, Tipton KD. Protein and amino acid metabolism during and after exercise and the effects of nutrition. Annu Rev Nutr 2000;20:457–83.
[16] Tarnopolsky M. Protein requirements for endurance athletes. Nutrition 2004;20:662–8.
[17] Tarnopolsky MA. Protein and physical performance. Curr Opin Clin Nutr Metab Care 1999;2:533–7.
[18] Tipton KD, Wolfe RR. Protein and amino acids for athletes. J Sports Sci 2004;22:65–79.
[19] Meredith CN, Zackin MJ, Frontera WR, et al. Dietary protein requirements and body protein metabolism in endurance-trained men. J Appl Physiol 1989;66:2850–6.
[20] Lamont LS, McCullough AJ, Kalhan SC. Comparison of leucine kinetics in endurance-trained and sedentary humans. J Appl Physiol 1999;86:320–5.
[21] Lamont LS, McCullough AJ, Kalhan SC. Relationship between leucine oxidation and oxygen consumption during steady-state exercise. Med Sci Sports Exerc 2001;33:237–41.
[22] McKenzie S, Phillips SM, Carter SL, et al. Endurance exercise training attenuates leucine oxidation and BCOAD activation during exercise in humans. Am J Physiol Endocrinol Metab 2000;278:E580–7.
[23] Phillips SM, Atkinson SA, Tarnopolsky MA, et al. Gender differences in leucine kinetics and nitrogen balance in endurance athletes. J Appl Physiol 1993;75:2134–41.
[24] Biolo G, Maggi SP, Williams BD, et al. Increased rates of muscle protein turnover and amino acid transport after resistance exercise in humans. Am J Physiol 1995;268: E514–20.
[25] Phillips SM, Tipton KD, Aarsland A, et al. Mixed muscle protein synthesis and breakdown following resistance exercise in humans. Am J Physiol Endocrinol Metab 1997;273: E99–107.
[26] Phillips SM, Tipton KD, Ferrando AA, et al. Resistance training reduces the acute exercise-induced increase in muscle protein turnover. Am J Physiol 1999;276:E118–24.
[27] Carraro F, Stuart CA, Hartl WH, et al. Effect of exercise and recovery on muscle protein synthesis in human subjects. Am J Physiol 1990;259:E470–6.
[28] Tipton KD, Ferrando AA, Williams BD, et al. Muscle protein metabolism in female swimmers after a combination of resistance and endurance exercise. J Appl Physiol 1996; 81:2034–8.
[29] Butterfield GE. Whole-body protein utilization in humans. Med Sci Sports Exerc 1987;19: S157–65.
[30] Todd KS, Butterfield GE, Calloway DH. Nitrogen balance in men with adequate and deficient energy intake at three levels of work. J Nutr 1984;114:2107–18.
[31] Millward DJ. Protein and amino acid requirements of athletes. J Sports Sci 2004;22: 143–4.
[32] Rennie MJ, Bohe J, Wolfe RR. Latency, duration and dose response relationships of amino acid effects on human muscle protein synthesis. J Nutr 2002;132:3225S–7S.

[33] Butterfield GE, Calloway DH. Physical activity improves protein utilization in young men. Br J Nutr 1984;51:171–84.
[34] Phillips SM, Parise G, Roy BD, et al. Resistance-training-induced adaptations in skeletal muscle protein turnover in the fed state. Can J Physiol Pharmacol 2002;80:1045–53.
[35] Hartman JW, Moore DR, Phillips SM. Resistance training reduces whole body protein turnover and improves net protein retention in untrained young males. Appl Physiol Nutr Metab 2006;31(5):557–64.
[36] Lamont LS, Patel DG, Kalhan SC. Leucine kinetics in endurance-trained humans. J Appl Physiol 1990;69:1–6.
[37] Lamont LS, McCullough AJ, Kalhan SC. Gender differences in leucine, but not lysine, kinetics. J Appl Physiol 2001;91:357–62.
[38] Anthony JC, Anthony TG, Layman DK. Leucine supplementation enhances skeletal muscle recovery in rats following exercise. J Nutr 1999;129:1102–6.
[39] Gautsch TA, Anthony JC, Kimball SR, et al. Availability of eIF4E regulates skeletal muscle protein synthesis during recovery from exercise. Am J Physiol 1998;274:C406–14.
[40] Sheffield-Moore M, Yeckel CW, Volpi E, et al. Postexercise protein metabolism in older and younger men following moderate-intensity aerobic exercise. Am J Physiol Endocrinol Metab 2004;287:E513–22.
[41] Sheffield-Moore M, Paddon-Jones D, Sanford AP, et al. Mixed muscle and hepatic derived plasma protein metabolism is differentially regulated in older and younger men following resistance exercise. Am J Physiol Endocrinol Metab 2005;288:E922–9.
[42] Deibert P, Konig D, Schmidt-Trucksaess A, et al. Weight loss without losing muscle mass in pre-obese and obese subjects induced by a high-soy-protein diet. Int J Obes Relat Metab Disord 2004;28:1349–52.
[43] Burke DG, Chilibeck PD, Davidson KS, et al. The effect of whey protein supplementation with and without creatine monohydrate combined with resistance training on lean tissue mass and muscle strength. Int J Sport Nutr Exerc Metab 2001;11:349–64.
[44] Nissen SL, Sharp RL. Effect of dietary supplements on lean mass and strength gains with resistance exercise: a meta-analysis. J Appl Physiol 2003;94:651–9.
[45] Millward DJ. Protein and amino acid requirements of adults: current controversies. Can J Appl Physiol 2001;26(Suppl):S130–40.
[46] Tome D, Bos C. Dietary protein and nitrogen utilization. J Nutr 2000;130:1868S–73S.
[47] Furst P, Stehle P. What are the essential elements needed for the determination of amino acid requirements in humans? J Nutr 2004;134:1558S–65S.
[48] Hegsted DM. Assessment of nitrogen requirements. Am J Clin Nutr 1978;31:1669–77.
[49] Young VR. Nutritional balance studies: indicators of human requirements or of adaptive mechanisms? J Nutr 1986;116:700–3.
[50] Young VR, Bier DM, Pellett PL. A theoretical basis for increasing current estimates of the amino acid requirements in adult man, with experimental support. Am J Clin Nutr 1989;50:80–92.
[51] Wolfe RR. Protein supplements and exercise. Am J Clin Nutr 2000;72:551S–7S.
[52] Millward DJ. Methodological considerations. Proc Nutr Soc 2001;60:3–5.
[53] Tipton KD. Gender differences in protein metabolism. Curr Opin Clin Nutr Metab Care 2001;4:493–8.
[54] Lemon PW. Protein and amino acid needs of the strength athlete. Int J Sport Nutr 1991;1: 127–45.
[55] Rennie MJ, Wackerhage H, Spangenburg EE, et al. Control of the size of the human muscle mass. Annu Rev Physiol 2004;66:799–828.
[56] Venderley AM, Campbell WW. Vegetarian diets: nutritional considerations for athletes. Sports Med 2006;36:293–305.
[57] Barr SI, Rideout CA. Nutritional considerations for vegetarian athletes. Nutrition 2004;20: 696–703.

[58] Janelle KC, Barr SI. Nutrient intakes and eating behavior scores of vegetarian and nonvegetarian women. J Am Diet Assoc. 1995;95:180–6 [quiz, 189].
[59] Rand WM, Pellett PL, Young VR. Meta-analysis of nitrogen balance studies for estimating protein requirements in healthy adults. Am J Clin Nutr 2003;77:109–27.
[60] Bos C, Juillet B, Fouillet H, et al. Postprandial metabolic utilization of wheat protein in humans. Am J Clin Nutr 2005;81:87–94.
[61] Fouillet H, Mariotti F, Gaudichon C, et al. Peripheral and splanchnic metabolism of dietary nitrogen are differently affected by the protein source in humans as assessed by compartmental modeling. J Nutr 2002;132:125–33.
[62] Morens C, Bos C, Pueyo ME, et al. Increasing habitual protein intake accentuates differences in postprandial dietary nitrogen utilization between protein sources in humans. J Nutr 2003;133:2733–40.
[63] Huang PC, Lin CP. Protein requirements of young Chinese male adults on ordinary Chinese mixed diet and egg diet at ordinary levels of energy intake. J Nutr 1982;112:897–907.
[64] Yanez E, Uauy R, Ballester D, et al. Capacity of the Chilean mixed diet to meet the protein and energy requirements of young adult males. Br J Nutr 1982;47:1–10.
[65] Yanez E, Uauy R, Zacarias I, et al. Long-term validation of 1 g of protein per kilogram body weight from a predominantly vegetable mixed diet to meet the requirements of young adult males. J Nutr 1986;116:865–72.
[66] Haub MD, Wells AM, Tarnopolsky MA, et al. Effect of protein source on resistive-training-induced changes in body composition and muscle size in older men. Am J Clin Nutr 2002;76:511–7.
[67] Calloway DH, Spector H. Nitrogen balance as related to caloric and protein intake in active young men. Am J Clin Nutr 1954;2:405–12.
[68] Pellett PL, Young VR. The effects of different levels of energy intake on protein metabolism and of different levels of protein intake on energy metabolism: a statistical evaluation from the published literature. In: Scrimshaw NS, Schurch B, editors. Protein-energy interactions. Lausanne (Switzerland): IDEGG, Nestle Foundation; 1992. p. 81–121.
[69] Chittenden RH. The nutrition of man. London: Heinemann; 1907.
[70] Rozenek R, Ward P, Long S, et al. Effects of high-calorie supplements on body composition and muscular strength following resistance training. J Sports Med Phys Fitness 2002;42:340–7.
[71] Gater DR, Gater DA, Uribe JM, et al. Impact of nutritional supplements and resistance training on body composition, strength and insulin-like growth factor-1. J Appl Sport Sci Res 1992;6:66–76.
[72] Boisseau N, Persaud C, Jackson AA, et al. Training does not affect protein turnover in pre- and early pubertal female gymnasts. Eur J Appl Physiol 2005;94:262–7.
[73] Lopez-Varela S, Montero A, Chandra RK, et al. Nutritional status of young female elite gymnasts. Int J Vitam Nutr Res 2000;70:185–90.
[74] Farnsworth E, Luscombe ND, Noakes M, et al. Effect of a high-protein, energy-restricted diet on body composition, glycemic control, and lipid concentrations in overweight and obese hyperinsulinemic men and women. Am J Clin Nutr 2003;78:31–9.
[75] Foster GD, Wyatt HR, Hill JO, et al. A randomized trial of a low-carbohydrate diet for obesity. N Engl J Med 2003;348:2082–90.
[76] Layman DK, Boileau RA, Erickson DJ, et al. A reduced ratio of dietary carbohydrate to protein improves body composition and blood lipid profiles during weight loss in adult women. J Nutr 2003;133:411–7.
[77] Layman DK, Evans E, Baum JI, et al. Dietary protein and exercise have additive effects on body composition during weight loss in adult women. J Nutr 2005;135:1903–10.
[78] Noakes M, Foster P, Keogh J, et al. Very low carbohydrate diets for weight loss and cardiovascular risk1. Asia Pac J Clin Nutr 2004;13:S64.
[79] Noakes M, Keogh JB, Foster PR, et al. Effect of an energy-restricted, high-protein, low-fat diet relative to a conventional high-carbohydrate, low-fat diet on weight loss, body

composition, nutritional status, and markers of cardiovascular health in obese women. Am J Clin Nutr 2005;81:1298–306.

[80] Layman DK, Walker DA. Potential importance of leucine in treatment of obesity and the metabolic syndrome. J Nutr 2006;136:319S–23S.

[81] Bolster DR, Jefferson LS, Kimball SR. Regulation of protein synthesis associated with skeletal muscle hypertrophy by insulin-, amino acid- and exercise-induced signalling. Proc Nutr Soc 2004;63:351–6.

[82] Kimball SR, Jefferson LS. Regulation of protein synthesis by branched-chain amino acids. Curr Opin Clin Nutr Metab Care 2001;4:39–43.

[83] Kimball SR, Jefferson LS. New functions for amino acids: effects on gene transcription and translation. Am J Clin Nutr 2006;83:500S–7S.

[84] Harber MP, Schenk S, Barkan AL, et al. Effects of dietary carbohydrate restriction with high protein intake on protein metabolism and the somatotropic axis. J Clin Endocrinol Metab 2005;90:5175–81.

[85] Bolster DR, Pikosky MA, Gaine PC, et al. Dietary protein intake impacts human skeletal muscle protein fractional synthetic rates following endurance exercise. Am J Physiol Endocrinol Metab 2005;289(4):E678–83.

[86] Koopman R, Wagenmakers AJ, Manders RJ, et al. Combined ingestion of protein and free leucine with carbohydrate increases postexercise muscle protein synthesis in vivo in male subjects. Am J Physiol Endocrinol Metab 2005;288:E645–53.

[87] Macdermid PW, Stannard SR. A whey-supplemented, high-protein diet versus a high-carbohydrate diet: effects on endurance cycling performance. Int J Sport Nutr Exerc Metab 2006;16:65–77.

[88] Quevedo MR, Price GM, Halliday D, et al. Nitrogen homoeostasis in man: diurnal changes in nitrogen excretion, leucine oxidation and whole body leucine kinetics during a reduction from a high to a moderate protein intake. Clin Sci (Lond) 1994;86:185–93.

[89] Bos C, Mahe S, Gaudichon C, et al. Assessment of net postprandial protein utilization of 15N-labelled milk nitrogen in human subjects. Br J Nutr 1999;81:221–6.

[90] Bos C, Metges CC, Gaudichon C, et al. Postprandial kinetics of dietary amino acids are the main determinant of their metabolism after soy or milk protein ingestion in humans. J Nutr 2003;133:1308–15.

[91] Dangin M, Boirie Y, Garcia-Rodenas C, et al. The digestion rate of protein is an independent regulating factor of postprandial protein retention. Am J Physiol Endocrinol Metab 2001;280:E340–8.

[92] Tipton KD, Elliott TA, Cree MG, et al. Ingestion of casein and whey proteins result in muscle anabolism after resistance exercise. Med Sci Sports Exerc 2004;36:2073–81.

[93] Fouillet H, Gaudichon C, Mariotti F, et al. Energy nutrients modulate the splanchnic sequestration of dietary nitrogen in humans: a compartmental analysis. Am J Physiol Endocrinol Metab 2001;281:E248–60.

[94] Gaudichon C, Mahe S, Benamouzig R, et al. Net postprandial utilization of [15N]-labeled milk protein nitrogen is influenced by diet composition in humans. J Nutr 1999;129: 890–5.

[95] Borsheim E, Tipton KD, Wolf SE, et al. Essential amino acids and muscle protein recovery from resistance exercise. Am J Physiol Endocrinol Metab 2002;283:E648–57.

[96] Borsheim E, Cree MG, Tipton KD, et al. Effect of carbohydrate intake on net muscle protein synthesis during recovery from resistance exercise. J Appl Physiol 2004;96:674–8.

[97] Borsheim E, Aarsland A, Wolfe RR. Effect of an amino acid, protein, and carbohydrate mixture on net muscle protein balance after resistance exercise. Int J Sport Nutr Exerc Metab 2004;14:255–71.

[98] Miller SL, Tipton KD, Chinkes DL, et al. Independent and combined effects of amino acids and glucose after resistance exercise. Med Sci Sports Exerc 2003;35:449–55.

[99] Biolo G, Williams BD, Fleming RY, et al. Insulin action on muscle protein kinetics and amino acid transport during recovery after resistance exercise. Diabetes 1999;48:949–57.

[100] Elliott TA, Cree MG, Sanford AP, et al. Milk ingestion stimulates net muscle protein synthesis following resistance exercise. Med Sci Sports Exerc 2006;38:667–80.
[101] Roy BD, Fowles JR, Hill R, et al. Macronutrient intake and whole body protein metabolism following resistance exercise. Med Sci Sports Exerc 2000;32:1412–8.
[102] Roy BD, Tarnopolsky MA, MacDougall JD, et al. Effect of glucose supplement timing on protein metabolism after resistance training. J Appl Physiol 1997;82:1882–8.
[103] Tipton KD, Rasmussen BB, Miller SL, et al. Timing of amino acid-carbohydrate ingestion alters anabolic response of muscle to resistance exercise. Am J Physiol Endocrinol Metab 2001;281:E197–206.
[104] Tipton KD, Elliot TA, Cree MG, et al. Stimulation of net muscle protein synthesis by whey protein ingestion before and after exercise. Am J Physiol, in press.
[105] Tipton KD, Borsheim E, Wolf SE, et al. Acute response of net muscle protein balance reflects 24-h balance after exercise and amino acid ingestion. Am J Physiol Endocrinol Metab 2003;284:E76–89.
[106] Paddon-Jones D, Sheffield-Moore M, Urban RJ, et al. Essential amino acid and carbohydrate supplementation ameliorates muscle protein loss in humans during 28 days bedrest. J Clin Endocrinol Metab 2004;89:4351–8.
[107] Pilegaard H, Ordway GA, Saltin B, et al. Transcriptional regulation of gene expression in human skeletal muscle during recovery from exercise. Am J Physiol Endocrinol Metab 2000;279:E806–14.
[108] Hargreaves M, Cameron-Smith D. Exercise, diet, and skeletal muscle gene expression. Med Sci Sports Exerc 2002;34:1505–8.
[109] Kimball SR, Farrell PA, Jefferson LS. Invited review: role of insulin in translational control of protein synthesis in skeletal muscle by amino acids or exercise. J Appl Physiol 2002;93: 1168–80.
[110] Hawley JA, Tipton KD, Millard-Stafford ML. Promoting training adaptations through nutritional interventions. J Sports Sci 2006;24:1–13.
[111] Pilegaard H, Osada T, Andersen LT, et al. Substrate availability and transcriptional regulation of metabolic genes in human skeletal muscle during recovery from exercise. Metabolism 2005;54:1048–55.
[112] Tipton KD, Sharp CP. The response of intracellular signaling and muscle protein metabolism to nutrition and exercise. Eur J Sports Sci 2005;5:107–21.
[113] Hargreaves M. Diet, genes and exercise performance. Asia Pac J Clin Nutr 2003; 12(Suppl):S1.
[114] Rasmussen BB, Tipton KD, Miller SL, et al. An oral essential amino acid-carbohydrate supplement enhances muscle protein anabolism after resistance exercise. J Appl Physiol 2000;88:386–92.

Clin Sports Med 26 (2007) 37–68
CLINICS IN SPORTS MEDICINE

ELSEVIER
SAUNDERS

Body Composition in Athletes: Assessment and Estimated Fatness

Robert M. Malina, PhD*
Tarleton State University, Stephenville, TX, USA

The study of body composition attempts to partition and quantify body weight or mass into its basic components. Body weight is a gross measure of the mass of the body, which can be studied at several levels from basic chemical elements and specific tissues to the entire body. Body composition is a factor that can influence athletic performance and as such is of considerable interest to athletes and coaches. This article provides an overview of models and methods used for studying body composition, changes in body composition during adolescence and the transition into adulthood, and applications to adolescent and young adult athletes.

LEVELS OF BODY COMPOSITION

The study of body composition historically has been driven by the availability of methods to measure or, more appropriately, to estimate it. Since the early 1980s, considerable progress has been made in the development and refinement of techniques to estimate the composition of the body, so that virtually all components of the body can now be measured. This progress has resulted in the modification of the models that provide the framework for studying body composition.

Body composition can be approached at a variety of levels. The five-level approach provides a sound guide: atomic, molecular, cellular, tissue, and whole body [1,2]. The multilevel view provides a framework within which the lure and difficulty inherent in the study of body composition can be appreciated.

Basic chemical elements compose the *atomic* level. There are 106 elements in nature. About 50 are found in the human body, and with more recent technologic advances, all 50 can be measured in vivo. Oxygen, carbon, hydrogen, and nitrogen account for greater than 95% of body mass, and the addition of seven other elements–sodium, potassium, phosphorus, chloride, calcium, magnesium, and sulfur–accounts for 99.5% of body mass [2].

The *molecular* level of body composition focuses on four of five components: water, lipid (fat), protein, minerals, and carbohydrate. The last component,

*10735 FM 2668 Bay City, TX 77414. *E-mail address:* rmalina@wcnet.net

0278-5919/07/$ – see front matter
doi:10.1016/j.csm.2006.11.004
© 2007 Elsevier Inc. All rights reserved.
sportsmed.theclinics.com

carbohydrate, occurs in small amounts in the form of glycogen, largely in the liver and skeletal muscle, and is not usually considered in estimates of body composition. The following equation is used:

$$\text{Body mass} = \text{water} + \text{protein} + \text{mineral} + \text{fat}$$

Most mineral is located in bone with a small fraction in other tissues. Historically, the relative contribution of each of the four components to body mass was derived from chemical analyses of human cadavers, although each can now be measured in vivo.

At the *cellular* level, body mass is viewed as composed of cells and substances outside of cells. The body cell mass (BCM) is defined by intracellular fluids and intracellular solids and is the metabolically active component of the body. Presently available methods do not permit measurement of cell solids in vivo. Extracellular fluids (ECF) and extracellular solids (ECS) compose the substances outside of the cells. The primary ECF are bone minerals and other components of connective tissues. Adipocytes are fat cells; they store lipids and comprise fat mass (FM). The equation is as follows:

$$\text{Body mass} = \text{BCM} + \text{ECF} + \text{ECS} + \text{FM}$$

At the *tissue* level, the study of body composition focuses on the contribution of specific tissues to body mass: skeletal muscle, adipose, bone, blood, viscera, and brain. Skeletal muscle, adipose, and bone tissues historically have been a primary focus in studies using traditional technologies, such as anthropometry and radiography. New technologies permit more refined assessment of these primary tissues (eg, the mineral content of bone tissue or subcutaneous versus internal adipose tissue).

The fifth level of body composition is the *whole body,* its size, shape, physique, and proportions. Anthropometry is the basic tool for estimating body size and configuration, although photographic techniques also have been used, especially for the study of shape and physique. The body mass index (BMI) (weight [kg]/height^2 [m]) and skinfold thicknesses are perhaps the most widely used anthropometric indicators at this level of body composition. Two other properties of the whole body are crucial in the study of body composition–volume and density.

MODELS OF BODY COMPOSITION

The two-component model historically has been the model of choice for partitioning body mass into meaningful components or compartments. This traditional approach has evolved into more complex models that include three, four, or more compartments.

Two Components

The two-component model partitions body mass into its lean (fat-free mass [FFM]) and fat (FM) compartments. The equation follows:

$$\text{Body mass} = \text{FFM} + \text{FM}$$

The term *lean body mass* is occasionally used, but FFM is more appropriate. Lean body mass is a more anatomic concept that includes some essential lipids, whereas FFM is a biochemical concept. This model has had the widest application in the study of body composition, including many studies of athletes. FM is the more labile of the two compartments; it is readily influenced by diet and training. A shortcoming of the two-component model is the heterogeneous composition of FFM; it includes water, protein, mineral (bone and soft tissue mineral), and glycogen.

Three Components

The three-component model includes FM and partitions FFM into total body water (TBW) and fat-free dry mass (FFDM). The equation is as follows:

$$\text{Body mass} = \text{TBW} + \text{FFDM} + \text{FM}$$

Water is the largest component of body mass, and most is located in lean tissues. FFDM includes protein, glycogen, and mineral in bone and soft tissues.

Four Components

With the development of techniques to measure bone mineral, the four-component model is a logical extension of the preceding model. FFDM is partitioned in bone mineral (BM) and the residual. The following equation is used:

$$\text{Body mass} = \text{TBW} + \text{BM} + \text{FM} + \text{residual}$$

Overview

All models include FM. It is the aspect of body composition that has received and continues to receive most attention. Excess FM can have a negative influence on physical performance and is often viewed by coaches and trainers as a major limiting factor in athletic achievements. Excessive fatness also is a major independent risk factor for several degenerative diseases.

FM, although often treated as a singular component of body composition, is heterogeneous. Fat, or more appropriately lipid, is physiologically divided into essential and nonessential lipids. Essential lipids are vital components of cells and are basic for a variety of physiologic functions; they constitute about 10% of total lipids in the body. The remaining lipids, 90% of total body lipids, are nonessential. They are triglycerides, which provide a storage form of available energy and perhaps thermal insulation [2]. The small amount of essential lipids in the body usually are not considered in estimates of body composition and usually are grouped with the residual component or with FM, depending on the model and method of assessment.

FFM is highly correlated with overall body size. Partitioning FFM into fractions has several problems. Error is inherent in the measurement of each component, and the more components included in a model increases the chances of error. The techniques available for the measurement of TBW, potassium, calcium, and sodium each have associated error. When measured, these properties must be converted to the body composition component of interest. The transformation of the measured property to the component is essentially mathematical and includes a variety of assumptions.

Multicomponent models are additive; it is assumed that the separately measured properties can be summed to provide an estimate of the whole. Thus, the measurement of body composition is essentially an estimate of body composition.

The different models of body composition have been largely developed on adults. They also assume that during periods of stable body mass, the various components exist in a steady state, which means that they are constant, or the relationships among components are constant. The assumption of constant relationships has permitted the development of procedures to estimate the different fractions of body mass in adults. The application of these procedures to children and adolescents, to adults in different stages of the life cycle, and to elite athletes requires care in interpretation of various estimates. The proportions of each component and the relationships among components change during growth and maturation and with aging. Systematic training for sport is an additional factor that influences body composition.

METHODS FOR ESTIMATING BODY COMPOSITION

Methods of estimating body composition in vivo are numerous and often quite complex (Table 1). The methods are sufficiently different in technique that one may inquire whether they provide reasonably similar estimates of body composition. The formulas for estimating FFM or FM, or components of FFM, and the assumptions underlying the procedures are based primarily on adults in the general population (ie, nonathletes). Their application to growing and maturing children and adolescents and to athletes may result in spuriously high or low estimates.

Several commonly used methods are briefly described. Three have been used regularly for some time–the measurement of body density (Db), TBW, and potassium concentration. Two more recent methods–dual-energy x-ray absorptiometry (DXA) and bioelectrical impedance analysis (BIA)–also are described. The specific protocols for each of these methods and their limitations are discussed in detail in Roche et al [3] and Heymsfield et al [4]. Anthropometric approaches also are briefly summarized.

Body Density—Densitometry

Density is mass per unit volume. The density of specific body tissues varies. The density of lean tissues ($\geq$1.100 g/cm^3) is greater than the density of water (1 g/cm^3) and fat (0.9007 g/cm^3). Density is inversely related to body fat

Table 1
Summary of methods used to estimate body composition

Method	Description
Underwater weighing, gas displacement	Estimates body density, which is converted to % Fat
Isotope dilution	Estimates total body water, which is converted to FFM; compartments of total body water also can be estimated
^{40}K whole-body counting	Estimates potassium content of body, which is converted to FFM
Dual-energy x-ray absorptiometry (DXA)	Estimates bone mineral, also lean and fat tissues
Bioelectrical impedance	Estimates FFM
Neutron activation analysis	Uses isotopes of nitrogen and calcium to estimate lean tissue and mineral
Uptake of fat-soluble gases	Estimates FM
24-hour urinary creatinine excretion	Estimates muscle mass
3-Methylhistidine excretion	Estimates muscle mass
MRI	Estimates of fat, muscle, and bone without ionizing radiation, plus chemical composition
CT	Estimates of bone, muscle, and fat
Ultrasound	Estimates of fat, muscle, and bone
Radiography	Estimates of fat, muscle, and bone
Anthropometry	Estimates of subcutaneous fat and predictions of FM and FFM

Data from Malina RM, Bouchard C, Bar-Or O. Growth, maturation, and physical activity. 2nd edition. Champaign (IL): Human kinetics; 2004.

content: The greater the proportion of fat, the lower the Db. A measure of Db permits an estimate of the percentage of body mass that is fat (% Fat).

The most common method for measuring Db is underwater (hydrostatic) weighing, but air or helium displacement techniques also are used. Two formulas are used most often to convert Db to % Fat:

$$\% \text{Fat} = 4.570/\text{Db} - 4.142 \ [5]$$

$$\% \text{Fat} = 4.950/\text{Db} - 4.500 \ [6]$$

The formulas and their underlying assumptions are derived from adults. The two equations give reasonably similar estimates of % Fat except for the very lean and very obese [7].

The estimate of % Fat is based on the assumption that the densities of the fat and fat-free components are known and are constant, and that adults are identical in composition except for variability in the proportion of fat. The proportions and chemical composition of the various components of FFM change with growth and maturation, in addition to interindividual differences in composition of FFM.

An estimate of FM is derived by multiplication and subtraction:

$$FM = \text{body mass} \times \%\,\text{Fat}$$

$$FFM = \text{body mass} - FM$$

Total Body Water—Hydrometry

Water is the largest component of the body, varying between 55% and 65% of body mass in normally hydrated young men, with lower values for women. The TBW of 70-kg young men can range from 38 to 45 kg of water. Emphasis is on normal hydration. TBW varies during the course of a day, depending on fluid intake and physical activity level, especially strenuous exercise. It also varies with severe protein-energy undernutrition and extreme obesity.

Most of the water in the body is in lean tissues. Water constitutes approximately 72% to 74% of FFM in normally hydrated adults, although the estimated water content of FFM has been reported to vary between 67% and 74%. In contrast, adipose tissue is relatively nonaqueous and contains a small proportion of water, about 20%.

The measurement of TBW provides an estimate of FFM. The process is based on two principles of isotope dilution: Certain substances distribute themselves evenly throughout a fluid space or compartment of the body, and the dilution of a known amount of substance, an isotope tracer, administered into an unknown volume or mass enables the calculation of the unknown volume or mass. The protocol consists of administering a known amount of a stable isotope tracer, allowing it sufficient time to dilute or mix, and then measuring its concentration after dilution and after correcting for the amount of the tracer lost from the body by excretion or exhalation. Three isotopes generally are used to measure TBW: deuterated water (^{2}H, deuterium), tritiated water (^{3}H, tritium), and ^{18}O-labeled water (heavy isotope of oxygen).

TBW usually is measured in the morning after an overnight fast. The isotope is administered to the subject based on body mass. Time is permitted for its equilibration with body water, usually 2 to 4 hours depending on the isotope. The concentration of the isotope in serum, urine, or saliva is measured. Assuming that the percentage of water in FFM is constant in adults, FFM is estimated as follows:

$$FFM = TBW/0.732$$

$$FM = \text{body mass} - FFM$$

TBW can be subdivided into water that is intracellular (ICW) and extracellular (ECW). Estimates of ICW and ECW in young men are 57% and 43% [8].

ECW usually is measured with the same isotope dilution principles as TBW with either chloride or bromide as the isotope. ECW is composed mainly of water in support and transport tissues: plasma, dense connective tissue (tendon, cartilage, bone), interstitial lymph, and transcellular fluids (cerebrospinal fluid, joint fluids). ICW corresponds closely to skeletal muscle mass, the work-producing tissue of the body, but is not exclusively composed of it. After estimating ECW, ICW usually is derived by subtraction:

$$\text{ICW} = \text{TBW} - \text{ECW}$$

Body Potassium—Whole Body Counting

Potassium occurs primarily in cells and especially in skeletal muscle tissue. Measurement of the concentration of potassium in the body can provide an estimate of FFM. This is done by measuring the amount of potassium-40 (^{40}K), a naturally occurring isotope of potassium that accounts for 0.0118% of the naturally occurring potassium in the human body [9]. The concentration of ^{40}K is measured with highly sensitive detection instruments, whole body counters, which count the gamma emissions of the naturally occurring potassium. A constant proportion of potassium in FFM is assumed, but there is a sex difference [10,11]. FFM is estimated as follows:

$$\text{FFM} = \text{mEq K}/68.1 \text{ in males}$$

$$\text{FFM} = \text{mEq K}/64.2 \text{ in females}$$

$$\text{FM} = \text{body mass} - \text{FFM}$$

More recent studies indicate variation in the potassium content of FFM, specifically values lower than the proportions indicated here [9]. Most of the available data for estimating body composition from measures of total body potassium use the constants reported by Forbes [10,11]. Total body potassium per unit FFM tends to decline with age in adulthood and shows differences between American blacks and whites [12,13].

Dual-Energy X-Ray Absorptiometry

DXA is used to measure bone mineral and soft tissue composition of the body. It provides estimates for the total body and of specific regions in the form of bone mineral, fat-free soft tissues (sometimes called bone-free lean tissue), and fat. The method requires a low radiation exposure, 0.05 to 1.5 mrem, depending on the machine and how quickly the total body scan is done [14]. The DXA unit measures the attenuation of the low-dose x-ray beam as it passes through different tissues of the body. How much of each photon beam is absorbed by the atoms in bone mineral and soft tissues of the body is recorded during the scan and converted to estimates of bone mineral and soft tissues [15]. The DXA instrument must be linked with appropriate computer algorithms to derive estimates of bone mineral, fat-free soft tissue, and fat tissue content of the total body. The algorithms also permit division of the body into anatomic segments–arms, legs, trunk, and head–to permit estimates of regional body composition.

The derivation of fat and fat-free soft tissue from DXA scans is based on the ratio of soft tissue attenuation of the low-energy and high-energy photon beams as they pass through the body. The attenuation of the low-energy and high-energy soft tissues is known based on scans of pure fat and fat-free soft tissues and theoretical calculations. It is assumed that the attenuation of fat and fat-free soft tissues is constant. The attenuation for fat is lower than that for fat-free soft tissues. Using these constants and the scans from the DXA unit, the amount of fat and fat-free soft tissue is calculated.

The derivation of bone mineral requires adjustment for the soft tissue overlying bone. DXA technology provides an estimate of total body bone mineral content (g) and total bone area (cm^3). The ratio of total body bone mineral to total bone area is used to estimate bone mineral density (g/cm^3). DXA basically measures the cross-sectional area of a scan (total bone area) and not bone volume; expressing bone mineral relative to bone area is only an approximation of bone mineral density.

Several types of commercially available DXA instruments are presently in use. Each type of unit has its own computer algorithms for deriving estimates of body composition, and there are inter-instrument differences. There is concern for the comparability of measurements, especially of soft tissue, from machines produced by different manufacturers. All of them assume that the attenuation characteristics of bone, fat-free soft tissue, and fat are known and constant [14].

Bioelectrical Impedance Analysis

The method of estimating body composition from BIA is based on the fact that lean tissue has a greater electrolyte and water content than fat. This difference in electrolyte content permits an estimate of FFM from the magnitude of the body's electrical conductivity or from the body's impedance to an electrical current as it flows from the source (usually the ankle) to the sink (usually the wrist) electrodes. FFM has low impedance and high conductivity, whereas FM, which has a relatively low water and electrolyte content, has high impedance and low conductivity.

BIA uses an imperceptible electrical current, which is introduced into the body via electrodes placed on the ankle. The injected current passes through the body, and the voltage that is produced is measured in voltage-sensing electrodes placed on the wrist [16,17]. The ratio of voltage to the current is impedance. Impedance to the flow of the current is related to the shape, volume, and length of the body, which is the conductor of the current. Because impedance is proportional to the geometry of the conductor, variation in body shape may be a factor in the application of BIA.

BIA measures the voltage for the path from the ankle to the wrist. It yields a measure of resistance, which is the major component of impedance. Resistance usually is converted to TBW, which is transformed into an estimate of FFM as described earlier. The equation used to convert resistance to TBW usually includes stature.

Several types of commercially available BIA units are presently in use, and there are differences among the units. They are portable (the size of a briefcase) and relatively inexpensive. BIA also is convenient, rapid, and noninvasive. As such, it is finding increased application for estimates of body composition. As with other methods, BIA has many underlying assumptions, which need to be verified.

Anthropometry

The use of anthropometric dimensions to estimate body composition has a long history [18,19]. Skinfold measurements are used most often to predict Db, which is converted to an estimate of % Fat. A variety of prediction equations incorporating skinfold measurements and other dimensions (height, limb and trunk circumferences, skeletal widths) are available. Most are based on samples of nonathlete adults, and several are based on children and adolescents, although equations for athletes also are available [19–23]. Prediction equations are sample specific and should be cross-validated. "Generalized" equations that adjust for age and the curvilinear relationship between skinfold thicknesses and Db also have been developed [24,25]. Equations based on advances in body composition methodology and multicomponent models also are available for the general population [26–28] and for female athletes [29].

Some degree of error is inherent in the measurement of body dimensions and body composition. Error associated with the measurements per se and with prediction equations should be noted. The standard error of estimate associated with available equations to predict body density generally ranges between 2% and 5%. For a discussion of error associated with anthropometry and the accuracy of body composition prediction equations, see Malina [30] and Sun and Chumlea [31].

More recently, the BMI has found increasing use as an alternative method for rapid assessment of body composition of athletes. The BMI is widely used in epidemiologic surveys of the weight status in adults: underweight (BMI <18.5 kg/m^2), overweight (BMI $\geq 25 < 30$ kg/m^2), and obesity (BMI ≥ 30 kg/m^2) [32]. It also is used as a screening device of overweight and obesity in children and adolescents [33,34]. The BMI is reasonably well correlated with total and percentage body fat in large and heterogeneous samples, although it has limitations especially with youth. Correlations between the BMI and FFM and FM are reasonably similar among youth, which would suggest that the BMI is an indicator of heaviness and indirectly of body fatness [35]. At the extremes of heaviness, the BMI is probably a reasonable indicator of fatness in the general population. Given the relatively large body size (height and mass) and relative leanness of athletes, the BMI has limitations with athletes.

Applications

The methods described provide an estimate of FFM and FM. Db is converted to % Fat; TBW, ^{40}K, and BIA (resistance) yield estimates of FFM. The other half of the two-component model is derived by subtraction. The three-component model involves the simultaneous measurement of Db and TBW to derive an estimate of % Fat, whereas the four-component model includes Db, TBW, and total body bone mineral to estimate % Fat. Multicomponent models provide the advantage of greater accuracy of estimates [36]. The cost and technical constraints of the required methodology often limit their applicability outside of the clinical or laboratory setting, however.

Most of the available body composition data for athletes are derived from the two-component model using Db. Data are less extensive for estimates derived from TBW, ^{40}K, multicomponent models, DXA, and BIA. The assumptions underlying the methods are based on nonathletic adults, and limitations of applications to youth and adult athletes need to be recognized. Fat estimates from densitometry are based on the assumption that the density of fat and lean tissues is constant. FFM estimates from TBW and ^{40}K are based on the assumption that the water and potassium contents of the FFM are constant. They also assume that the density of fat and lean tissues and the water and potassium contents of the FFM are the same in children, adolescents, and adults, which is not the case. An important issue in growing and maturing individuals is the age at which adult density, water concentration, and potassium concentration of FFM are achieved (see later).

BIA is finding increased application. The method is useful to describe the body composition of groups, but estimates have large errors within individuals, which limits its application. BIA is influenced by nutritional and hydration status and is not sensitive to acute changes in electrolytes and fluids. There also is significant variation between BIA machines produced by different manufacturers. The resistance (R) function of impedance is used most often with stature (length of the conductor) to estimate FFM, but there is uncertainty about the appropriate hydration factor to use in converting R to FFM. Other equations use R and stature, in conjunction with body mass, circumferences, and skinfold measurements to estimate FFM.

DXA is used most often to estimate bone mineral content and density. DXA measures of total body bone mineral content also are used in the four-component model to increase the accuracy of body composition estimates. The procedures require the measurement of Db, TBW, and bone mineral, and it is unclear whether the time and expense involved markedly improve the accuracy of the body composition estimates.

DXA also is being used more often to estimate FFM, FM, and % Fat. The accuracy of these estimates needs further verification relative to estimates derived from the more established methods of body composition assessment, specifically densitometry and hydrometry.

An important issue in all body composition studies is validation. How accurately does a given technique estimate the specific components of body composition? What is the appropriate criterion against which to compare estimates of body composition derived from the different methods and models? Do the different methods and models provide the same estimates of FFM, FM, and % Fat? The assessment of bone mineral content increases the accuracy of the four-component model over the three-component model. The instrument to measure bone mineral content is expensive, however: Is this expense justifiable given the small increase in the accuracy of the body composition estimates? These and other questions need to be considered in evaluating the application of new technologies and multicomponent models.

CHEMICAL MATURITY

If the principles and methods for estimating body composition are to be accurately applied to youth, including young athletes, it is important to determine when during growth are adult values for the primary components of FFM attained. When adult values are reached, chemical maturity is said to be attained. The concept of chemical maturity was introduced by Moulton [37]: "The point at which the concentration of water, proteins, and salts [minerals] becomes comparatively constant in the fat-free cell is named the point of chemical maturity of the cell."

During the interval of growth and maturation, approximately the first 2 decades of life, the relative contribution of water to body mass decreases, and corresponding contributions of solids–protein, mineral, and fat–to body mass increase. Growth is an accretive process, adding or accumulating solids at the expense of fluids. The relative contributions of protein and mineral to FFM also increase, whereas the relative contribution of water to FFM decreases.

The estimated composition of FFM from late childhood through adolescence into young adulthood is summarized in Table 2. With growth and maturation during adolescence, the relative contribution of solids (protein and mineral) to FFM increases, and that of water decreases. Sex differences are apparent. FFM in males contains relatively less water and relatively more protein and mineral compared with females. The sex difference also is reflected in the estimated potassium content and density of the FFM, which are greater in males than in females. The difference reflects the sex difference in muscle mass and bone mineral and persists into young adulthood. The gain in bone mineral between age 10 years and young adulthood reflects, to a large extent, the growth and maturation of the skeleton during the adolescent growth spurt. The relative mineral content of FFM in males increases from 5.4% at about 10 years to 6.6% at 17 to 20 years, a small increment (1.2%) that is, however, about 22% of the initial value at age 10. The corresponding increase in the relative mineral content of FFM in females is less, 5.2% to 6.1%, a relative increase

Table 2
Estimated composition of the Fat-free mass during the transition into adolescence, adolescence, and young adulthood

Age (y)	Compartments of the FFM (%)			Potassium (g/kg)	Density (g/cm^3)
	Water	Protein	Mineral		
Males					
9–11	76.2	18.4	5.4	2.45	1.084
11–13	75.4	18.9	5.7	2.52	1.087
13–15	74.7	19.1	6.2	2.56	1.094
15–17	74.2	19.3	6.5	2.61	1.096
17–20	74.0	19.4	6.6	2.63	1.099
Females					
9–11	77.0	17.8	5.2	2.34	1.082
11–13	76.6	17.9	5.5	2.36	1.086
13–15	75.5	18.6	5.9	2.38	1.092
15–17	75.0	18.9	6.1	2.40	1.094
17–20	74.8	19.2	6.0	2.41	1.095

The protein content of the FFM in the estimates is derived by subtraction: 100 – water – mineral = protein.
Data from Lohman TG. Applicability of body composition techniques and constants for children and youths. Exerc Sport Sci Rev 1986;14:325–57.

of about 16% of the initial value in late childhood. It is apparent that chemical maturity of FFM is not attained until after the adolescent growth spurt, probably about 16 to 18 years in girls and 18 to 20 years in boys.

The information summarized in Table 2 represents *estimates* of the chemical composition of the FFM. The estimates are derived in part from limited biochemical cadaver analyses and from in vivo estimates of TBW, potassium, nitrogen, calcium, and bone mineral. Estimates also vary from laboratory to laboratory, which is not unexpected because different data, assumptions, and methods are used in their derivation. There are continued efforts to arrive at the more accurate estimates of the chemical composition of the FFM. Nevertheless, an important conclusion to be derived from these estimates and ongoing studies is that the chemical maturity of FFM changes during growth and maturation and is not attained until late adolescence or young adulthood. The equations and constants based on adult values and earlier studies are often adjusted for the chemical immaturity of the FFM in growing and maturing individuals.

CHANGES IN BODY DENSITY, TOTAL BODY WATER, AND TOTAL BODY POTASSIUM DURING GROWTH

The basic properties used for estimating body composition change with growth and maturation [35,38,39]. TBW and total body potassium, both of which are found primarily in lean tissue, follow a growth pattern similar to that of height and body mass with a clear adolescent spurt during which growth in TBW and total body potassium is greater in males than in females. Both reach a plateau at about 15 to 17 years in females and increase into the early 20s in males. Db has a different growth pattern. It declines in males from about 8 to 10 years, but then increases more or less linearly to about 16 to 17 years of age. In females, Db decreases from about 8 to 11 years, then increases only slightly, and finally reaches a plateau by about 14 years. Both sexes also show a slight decline in Db in late adolescence and young adulthood. Db is inversely related to body fat content, although not linearly. Males have greater Db than females at all ages and have a correspondingly lower % Fat.

GROWTH IN FAT-FREE MASS, FAT MASS, AND FAT PERCENTAGE OF BODY MASS

The growth patterns of FFM, FM, and % Fat from late childhood through adolescence into young adulthood have been described [35]. FFM follows a growth pattern similar to that of height and weight. Sex differences are small during childhood and become established during the adolescent growth spurt. Young adult values of FFM are reached earlier in females, about 15 to 16 years, compared with 19 to 20 years in males. In late adolescence and young adulthood, males have, on average, an FFM that is about 1.5 times larger than that of females. The average FFM of young women is about 70% of the mean value for men. The difference reflects the male adolescent spurt in muscle mass and the sex difference in adult height.

When FFM is expressed per unit height (kg/cm), the sex difference is relatively small in late childhood and early adolescence, but after 14 years of age, males have more FFM for the same height as females. The sex difference increases with age so that young men have an estimated 0.36 kg FFM/cm height, whereas young women have an estimated 0.26 kg FFM/cm height.

Estimated FM increases more rapidly in females than in males from late childhood through adolescence, but seems to reach a plateau or to change only slightly near the time of the adolescent growth spurt in boys (about 13–15 years). In contrast to FFM, females have, on average, about 1.5 times the FM of males in late adolescence and young adulthood.

Estimated % Fat is greater in females than in males from late childhood through adolescence into young adulthood. Percent Fat increases gradually through adolescence in the same manner as FM in females; it also increases gradually in males until just before the adolescent spurt (about 11–12 years) and then gradually declines. Percent Fat reaches its lowest point at about 16 to 17 years in males and then gradually increases into young adulthood. In contrast to estimates of FM, % Fat declines during male adolescence. The decline is due to the rapid growth of FFM and slower accumulation of FM at this time. As such, fat contributes a lesser percentage to body mass in male adolescence.

To illustrate the impact of adolescence on body composition, differences in estimates of body composition between early and late adolescence are summarized in Table 3. Corresponding data for a mixed-longitudinal sample of youth from the Fels Longitudinal Study are included for comparison [40]. The Fels data are derived from subjects who had at least six serial measurements of Db between 8 and 23 years. A multicomponent model that included

Table 3
Estimated differences in densitometric estimates of body composition from early to late adolescence

	Males	Females
Composite sample[a]		
FFM	32.5 kg	17.3 kg
FM	3.2 kg	7.1 kg
% Fat	−2.7%	+5.0%
Fels sample[b]		
FFM	31.3 kg	14.0 kg
FM	3.4 kg	7.4 kg
% Fat	−3.5%	+3.8%

[a]*Adapted from* Malina et al. [39] and Malina [38], compiled from the literature. Estimates are differences between 10–11 and 18–19 years.
[b]Estimated from Guo et al. [40], mixed-longitudinal data. Estimates are the differences between two age groups, 10–12 and 18–20 years.

age-specific and sex-specific estimates of the density and major components of FFM was used to derive % Fat, FM, and FFM [40]. Allowing for methodologic variation, the estimates are reasonably similar. Males gain almost twice as much FFM as females over adolescence, and females gain about twice as much FM as males. The net result is a decline in relative fatness in males and an increase in relative fatness in females.

A major portion of changes in body composition over adolescence is concentrated in the interval of rapid growth in height. Peak height velocity (PHV) occurs, on average, at 12 and 14 years of age in a sample of North American and European girls and boys [35]. Assuming 1 year each side of PHV, the interval between 11 and 13 years in girls and 13 and 15 years in boys provides an estimate of changes in body composition at this time (Table 4). The interval of maximal growth in height accounts for about 40% of the total adolescent gain in FFM and FM. Although these estimates are based on cross-sectional data from the literature, they correspond reasonably well with limited data from longitudinal studies. Czech boys, many of whom were athletes, gained

Table 4
Estimated changes in FFM, FM and % Fat during the interval of maximal growth in height during the adolescent spurt[a]

	Total gain/loss		Annual gain/loss	
	Females	Males	Females	Males
FFM	7.1 kg	14.3 kg	3.5 kg/yr	7.2 kg/yr
FM	2.8 kg	1.5 kg	1.4 kg/yr	0.7 kg/yr
% Fat	1.7%	−1.1%	0.9%/yr	−0.5%/yr

Based on the composite data summarized in Table 2.
[a]Adolescent spurt: ~11–13 years in girls and ~13–15 years in boys.

about 7.5 kg/y in FFM and 0.8 kg/y in FM and declined about 0.4%/y in % Fat near the time of PHV [41]. The decline in relative fatness is an effect of the larger increase in FFM, so that FM, although increasing slightly, contributes a small percentage of body mass at this time. In the mixed-longitudinal sample from the Fels study (see Table 2), peak gain in FFM was about 7 kg/y in boys, whereas no clear spurt in FFM was evident in girls [40]. In a separate analysis of adolescent changes in total body bone mineral content, peak gains occurred, on average, a bit more than one half of a year after PHV in both sexes. Estimated peak gain in BMC was, on average, greater in boys, 407 ± 93 g/y, than in girls, 325 ± 67 g/y [42]. Peak gain in bone mineral content occurred closer to the age of menarche, suggesting that adolescent growth in bone mineral is closely related to sexual maturation in girls [42].

BODY COMPOSITION OF ATHLETES

Why Estimate the Body Composition of Athletes?

It is important to know how the different components of body composition vary with age, sex, and maturity status, especially during adolescence. Likewise, it is important to understand the influence of systematic training for sport on body composition. Many discussions of body composition in athletes focus on relative fatness because of the potentially negative influence of excessive fatness on performance. Focus of such discussions is often on female athletes, usually in the context of low levels of fatness, late sexual maturation, menstrual irregularities, and disordered eating. Weight control and in many instances reduction are issues with many athletes. Associated concerns are potential metabolic complications with long-term weight reduction [23] and weight control behaviors that may lead to complications of disordered eating, particularly among female athletes. Among male athletes, there is concern for low levels of fatness of males in weight category sports, specifically wrestling.

Youth Athletes

The body composition of young athletes is influenced by their growth and maturity status. With few exceptions, young athletes of both sexes tend to be at or above median reference values in height and mass; exceptions are gymnasts of both sexes and female figure skaters. Elite young male athletes tend to be, on average, advanced in maturity status, although there is variation among sports. Earlier maturation in males is associated with larger size and FFM, greater strength and power, and a lower % Fat compared with average ("on time") and later maturing peers of the same chronologic age. The size, strength, and power associated with earlier maturation in males are an advantage in many sports. Elite young female athletes tend to be, on average, average and later in maturity status compared with peers of the same chronologic age. Later maturation in females is associated with smaller body size, a more linear physique, lower % Fat, and generally better performances compared with early maturing peers [35]. Discussions of the body composition of young athletes should consider individual differences in maturity status; studies rarely consider maturity-association variation among young athletes. Variation associated with individual differences in biologic maturation is a potential confounding factor in evaluating the body composition of young athletes.

Because FFM follows a growth pattern similar to that for height and mass, and FFM is highly correlated with height and mass, most studies of body composition of young athletes emphasize % Fat. As noted, excessive fatness tends to exert a negative influence on performances, especially performances that require the movement or projection of the body through space (ie, running, jumping, vaulting), in contrast to those that require projection of objects (ie, shot put, discus throw). Coaches of young athletes often focus on weight control and relative fatness. Middle school, high school, and collegiate wrestling currently set minimum weight or % Fat requirements (see later).

Estimates of the relative fatness of adolescent athletes in a variety of sports are shown relative to data for nonathletes in Fig. 1. The estimates are means based on densitometry with one exception; data for a sample of female gymnasts based on DXA also are included. Allowing for variation among samples and in methodology, athletes as a rule have a lower % Fat than nonathletes of the same chronologic age. Male athletes and nonathletes show a decrease in % Fat during adolescence; athletes have less relative fatness at most ages, but there is considerable overlap (Fig. 1A). In contrast, % Fat in female athletes tends to be reasonably stable across adolescence, whereas that for nonathletes increases with age (Fig. 1B). The difference in % Fat between female athletes

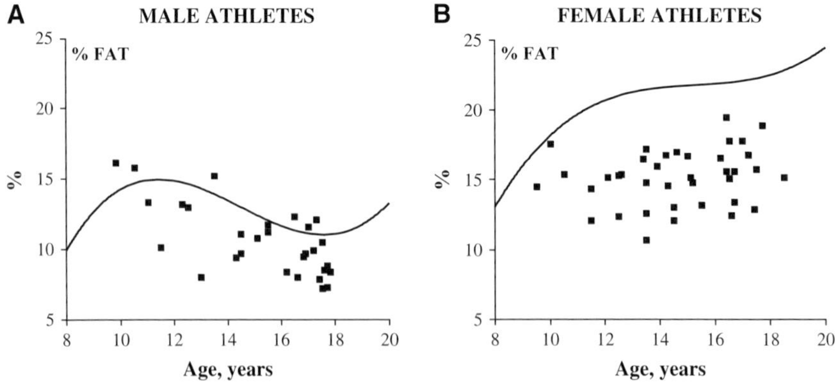

Fig. 1. Estimates of % Fat in samples of youth athletes. (*A*) Males. (*B*) Females. Male athletes include cyclists, wrestlers, gymnasts, runners, jumpers, and volleyball, ice hockey, and American football players. Female athletes include swimmers, runners, jumpers, gymnasts, and speed skaters. (See ref. [35] for sources of data. Data for the nonathlete reference from Malina et al [35,39].)

and nonathletes is greater than that between male athletes and nonathletes. Allowing for the sports represented, there seems to be more variation in % Fat among female than male athletes 14 to 18 years old.

Young Adult Athletes

Estimated % Fat in young adult male and female athletes in numerous sports is summarized in Tables 5 and 6. Most data are based on body density derived from hydrostatic weighing; estimates based on other methods are limited. Data for youth and adult track and field athletes by discipline are considered separately (see later).

The data summarized in Tables 5 and 6 provide an overview of estimated relative fatness and associated variation in young adult athletes in a variety of sports. Samples sizes are generally small, and many sports are not well represented. Corresponding estimates for % Fat predicted from skinfold measurements in national-level Polish athletes [43] and American intercollegiate female athletes in numerous sports are summarized in Tables 7 and 8, respectively. Within corresponding sports, % Fat of female athletes is, on average, greater than that of male athletes. Variation in % Fat by position or event within a sport is apparent for American football players (see Table 5), but is not marked among female basketball, volleyball, and track and field athletes, with the exception of the throwing events (Table 8).

The ethnic composition of samples of athletes is not usually reported; this is relevant given ethnic variation in body proportions and composition [13]. Ethnic variation in bone mineral content between American blacks and whites has been long documented [13] and influences estimates of Db via hydrostatic weighing [44]. Observations using more recent technology indicate that black women have a larger appendicular skeletal muscle mass than white women matched for age, body size, and menstrual status [45,46]. The ethnic difference is more marked in the upper than the lower extremity [45]. Limited data for American black and white males show less ethnic variation in limb musculature, but after adjustment for age, height, and mass, skeletal muscle mass of the legs is significantly larger in American blacks of both sexes. The ethnic difference also persists after adjusting for variation in relative leg length. Arm skeletal muscle mass also is significantly larger in American blacks of both sexes after adjusting for age and mass and for relative arm length [47].

The preceding observations on ethnic variation are based on nonathletes. Corresponding body composition data for athletes are limited. Estimated fatness (hydrostatic weighing) of collegiate football players is lower in black (14.7 ± 5.6%, $n = 55$) than white (19.0 ± 7.1%, $n = 35$) players [48]. Relative fatness estimated from skinfold measurements gives similar estimates, but BIA tends to overestimate % Fat based on Db, and near-infrared spectrophotometry tends to underestimate % Fat based on Db in black and white players [48]. Among female collegiate athletes, differences in estimated % Fat predicted from skinfold measurements between black and white athletes are, on average,

Table 5
Relative fatness (% Fat) in samples of male athletes in several sports

Sport	Age (y)			% Fat			Reference
	n	Mean	SD	Method	Mean	SD	
Badminton	7	24.5	3.6	HW	12.8	3.1	[21]
Baseball	10	20.8	9.9	TBW	14.2	6.7	[69]
Basketball	10	20.9	1.3	HW	10.5	3.8	[62]
Basketball	11	25.7	3.1	HW	9.7	3.1	[21]
Canoeing/kayaking	19	21.1	7.1	HW	13.0	2.5	[65]
Cycling	11	22.2	3.6	HW	10.5	2.4	[21]
Cycling	11	21.7	1.7	TBW	13.7	2.3	[66]
Cycling	13	24.1	3.1	HW	11.2	3.3	[67]
Cycling	63	21.9	3.2	HW	11.8	3.3	[65]
Field hockey	14	23.7	3.6	HW	10.3	4.4	[21]
Football by modality							
American football	21	19.9		^{40}K	9.5		[68]
American football	16	20.3	0.9	TBW	13.8	6.7	[69]
American football	65	17–23		HW	15.0	5.8	[70]
Defensive back	15			HW	11.5	2.7	
Offensive back, receiver	15			HW	12.4	5.3	
Defensive lineman	15			HW	18.5	4.4	
Defensive linebacker	7			HW	13.4	4.1	
Offensive lineman	13			HW	19.1	7.0	
American football							[71]
Defensive back	26	24.5	3.2	HW	9.6	4.2	
Offensive back, receiver	40	24.7	3.0	HW	9.4	4.0	
Quarterback, kicker	16	24.1	2.7	HW	14.4	6.5	
Defensive lineman	32	25.7	3.4	HW	18.2	5.4	
Defensive linebacker	28	24.2	2.4	HW	14.0	4.6	
Offensive lineman	38	24.7	3.2	HW	15.6	3.8	
American football, blacks	55	19.4	1.2	HW	14.7	5.6	[48]
American football, whites	35	19.7	1.5	HW	19.0	7.1	[48]
Australian rules	23	24.5	4.3	HW	8.0	3.0	[21]
Rugby union	16	24.2	3.3	HW	10.3	3.2	[21]
Soccer	9	24.8	1.9	TBW	6.2	1.9	[72]
Soccer	18	26.0	—	HW	9.6	—	[73]
Soccer	22	24.5	3.5	HW	6.9	3.3	[74]
Soccer	12	25.3	4.0	HW	9.7	3.0	[21]
Gymnastics	7	20.3	0.9	TBW	4.6	3.3	[69]
Gymnastics	8	20.2	2.7	HW	7.9	1.4	[21]
Ice hockey	27	24.9	3.6	HW	9.2	4.6	[75]
Lacrosse	26	26.7	4.2	HW	12.3	4.3	[21]
Rowing	8	24.7	3.2	TBW	7.3	1.3	[72]
Rowing	7	24.7	1.9	HW	11.2	1.4	[21]

(continued on next page)

Table 5
(continued)

	Age (y)			% Fat			
Sport	*n*	Mean	SD	Method	Mean	SD	Reference
Skiing	9	25.9	2.9	HW	6.3	1.9	[76]
Skiing, cross-country	11	22.8	1.9	HW	7.2	1.9	[75]
Skiing, cross-country	11	24.0	4.5	HW	12.3	4.6	[65]
Speed skating	33	18.4	2.9	HW	11.2	2.8	[65]
Speed skating	6	22.2	4.1	HW	7.4	2.5	[78]
Squash	9	22.6	6.8	HW	11.2	3.7	[21]
Swimming	7	20.6	1.2	TBW	5.0	4.5	[69]
Swimming	13	21.8	2.2	HW	8.5	2.9	[76]
Swimming	14	19.9	2.3	TBW	7.5	3.0	[72]
Swimming	39	19.1	4.5	HW	12.3	4.6	[65]
Volleyball	19	23.8	3.2	HW	11.2	2.8	[65]
Volleyball	11	20.9	3.7	HW	9.8	2.9	[21]
Water polo	10	25.8	4.6	TBW	8.8	2.6	[72]

Abbreviations: HW, hydrostatic weighing; TBW, total body water; ^{40}K, potassium 40.

quite small (see Table 8) and within the range of error associated with the prediction equation [49].

Adolescent and Young Adult Track and Field Athletes

Data on the size, physique, and body composition of track and field athletes in specific events within the sport are more extensive compared with other sports and span early adolescence through young adulthood. The literature dealing with track and field athletes is diverse and can be summarized in the framework of four general themes: (1) talent identification and selection; (2) interest in the growth, body composition, and functional characteristics of elite young athletes in a variety of sports; (3) increased popularity of distance running for children and adolescents; and (4) interest in the comparative morphology of athletes in general. The data often include estimates of % Fat based primarily on measured Db and predicted Db based on skinfold measurements; estimates based on other methods are limited [50]. The data permit evaluation of variation in % Fat by event. Estimates of mean % Fat are summarized in Figs. 2, 3, and 4 for sprinters and hurdlers, middle and long distance runners, and jumpers and throwers. Corresponding estimates for specific jumping and throwing disciplines, pole vaulters, race walkers, and decathletes are not extensive. Data for adolescents and young adults from the general population are included for comparison.

Most samples of male sprinters and hurdlers tend to be below the reference in % Fat from early adolescence into young adulthood, although there is some overlap during adolescence (Fig. 2A). In contrast, % Fat of female sprinters and hurdlers is well below the reference (Fig. 2B).

Estimates of % Fat among middle and long distance runners show considerable overlap within sex, although there seems to be more variation among

Table 6
Relative fatness (% Fat) in samples of female athletes in several sports

	Age (y)			% Fat			
Sport	*n*	Mean	SD	Method	Mean	SD	Reference
Badminton	6	23.0	5.3	HW	21.0	2.1	[22]
Basketball	18	22.9	2.6	HW	20.1	4.0	[22]
Canoeing/kayaking	21	21.2	3.7	HW	22.2	4.6	[65]
Field hockey	13	19.8	1.4	HW	21.3	7.1	[79]
Field hockey	17	22.6	2.3	HW	20.2	6.0	[22]
Field hockey	10	19.8	1.2	DXA	18.3	2.7	[80]
Gymnastics	5	19.0	3.8	TBW	12.9	1.4	[81]
Gymnastics	44	19.4	1.1	HW	15.3	4.0	[82]
Gymnastics	15	19.8	1.0	DXA	19.1	2.2	[80]
Gymnastics, rhythmic	7	20.7	2.7	HW	15.6	5.1	[65]
Handball, team	17	23.2	1.9	HW	19.0	3.7	[65]
Lacrosse	17	24.4	4.5	HW	19.3	5.7	[22]
Netball	7	23.7	4.2	HW	17.8	3.8	[22]
Rowing	19	23.6	3.9	HW	18.4	3.9	[65]
Rowing	22	20.4	1.9	DXA	21.9	2.3	[80]
Rowing, lightweight	5	19.4	7.5	HW	20.7	3.1	[22]
Rowing, heavyweight	7	20.5	3.4	HW	24.2	4.2	[22]
Skiing, cross country	5	23.5	4.7	HW	16.1	1.6	[77]
Soccer	10	24.4	4.5	HW	20.8	4.7	[83]
Soccer	11	22.1	4.1	HW	22.0	6.8	[22]
Soccer	10	19.8	0.9	DXA	21.8	2.7	[80]
Softball	14	22.6	4.0	HW	19.1	5.0	[22]
Softball	17	20.4	1.4	DXA	20.9	3.9	[80]
Speed skating	9	19.7	3.0	HW	16.5	4.1	[78]
Squash	6	27.4	5.6	HW	16.0	4.9	[22]
Swimming	19	19.2	0.8	HW	16.1	3.7	[20]
Tennis	7	21.3	0.9	HW	22.4	2.0	[79]
Volleyball	36	21.7	2.5	HW	15.8	4.8	[65]
Volleyball	13	23.0	2.6	HW	11.7	3.7	[84]
Volleyball	13	21.5	0.7	HW	18.3	3.4	[84]
Volleyball	11	22.8	3.4	HW	17.0	3.3	[22]

Abbreviations: HW, hydrostatic weighing; TBW, total body water.

females than males (Fig. 3). Most estimates for males are below the reference during adolescence into young adulthood (Fig. 3A). The reported estimate for a sample of 17-year-old male distance runners (2.6%) is spuriously low. As noted, % Fat of female middle distance and distance runners varies (Fig. 3B). Most values are below the reference value, but several approach the reference in later adolescence. In young adulthood, however, estimates of % Fat are considerably lower, especially in distance runners.

Estimated % Fat of field athletes in jumping and throwing events shows two distributions with little overlap (Fig. 4). The relative fatness of male jumpers is consistently below the reference from adolescence into adulthood. In contrast, % Fat of male adolescent throwers is consistently above the reference, reflecting

Table 7
Anthropometric estimates of predicted relative fatness (% Fat) in national level Polish athletes 19–26 years old

	Males	% Fat		Females	% Fat	
Sport	*n*	Mean	SD	*n*	Mean	SD
Basketball	24	10.4	2.5	31	20.1	4.8
Biathlon	10	10.8	2.0	10	17.2	3.9
Cycling	29	11.6	1.4	—	—	—
Fencing	21	12.0	3.4	15	21.9	4.5
Handball, team	23	12.7	3.1	29	21.9	4.7
Kayaking	29	9.6	2.7	26	16.3	4.3
Rowing	31	10.7	3.0	22	17.7	3.8
Skiing	13	9.6	1.5	10	17.0	1.8
Soccer	30	9.7	2.1	—	—	—
Swimming	—	—	—	13	15.5	2.5
Tennis	—	—	—	7	17.7	1.5
Volleyball	26	10.8	1.7	—	—	—

Relative fatness was estimated from predicted Db using three skinfolds after Piechaczek [85].

Data from Krawczyk B, Sklad M, Majle B. Body components of male and female athletes representing various sports. Biol Sport 1995;12:243–50.

in part their massiveness. Percent Fat tends to decline with age, however, among samples of throwers. Among young adult throwers, estimates for several samples are lower than corresponding values for adolescent throwers and fluctuate above and below the reference values (Fig. 4A).

Female jumpers have relative fatness levels consistently below the reference, and % Fat in young adult jumpers tends to be lower than that for adolescents (Fig. 4B). Percent Fat of female throwers varies above and below the reference in adolescence and young adulthood, which is in contrast to the trend in male throwers. In female jumpers and throwers, variation in % Fat is greater among young adults than among adolescents.

Estimates of % Fat in male track and field athletes except for throwers are generally below the reference. There is considerable overlap among mean estimates for sprinters and hurdlers, middle distance and distance runners, and jumpers, and all have % Fat that is generally lower than in samples of throwers. Trends in % Fat among adolescent track and field athletes should be viewed in two contexts: first, the decline in % Fat that accompanies the growth spurt and sexual maturation in males, and second, the decline in % Fat associated with systematic training [35].

In female track and field athletes, there is considerable overlap in mean estimates of % Fat among for runners of all disciplines and jumpers, and all are, on average, generally below the reference. Relative fatness of female throwers tends to be higher, but estimates fall above and below the reference.

Comparison of % Fat of male and female athletes within the same track and field events suggests several trends: (1) Percent Fat in male sprinters and

Table 8
Anthropometric estimates of predicted relative fatness (% Fat) in female university athletes by sport, event/position, and ethnicity

Sport	Age (y)			% Fat	
	n	Mean	SD	Mean	SD
Swimming	87	18.8	0.9	16.5	1.6
Freestyle	37	18.8	0.8	16.3	1.6
Backstroke	18	18.9	1.0	16.8	1.9
Breaststroke	17	18.7	0.7	16.4	1.3
Butterfly	9	19.1	1.0	16.4	1.9
Medley	6	18.9	1.4	17.5	0.8
Diving	19	19.5	1.6	17.4	2.6
Tennis	29	19.0	0.9	17.7	2.4
Golf	32	19.0	0.9	19.1	2.2
Basketball	57	19.5	1.2	16.4	2.2
Guard, white	13	19.4	0.9	16.9	2.1
Guard, black	7	19.6	1.2	14.9	1.2
Wing, white	6	19.3	0.9	16.1	1.4
Wing, black	11	19.8	1.5	15.5	1.7
Post, white	11	19.6	1.4	17.4	3.0
Post, black	9	19.6	1.6	17.1	2.5
Volleyball	47	19.1	0.9	16.9	2.7
Outside hitter	24	19.2	1.0	16.9	3.0
Middle blocker	12	18.7	0.7	17.8	2.6
Setter	6	19.2	0.8	17.0	1.9
Back row	5	19.2	0.5	14.9	1.3
Track and field	116	19.4	1.2	15.4	3.8
Sprint, white	5	21.1	1.4	14.1	0.3
Sprint, black	38	19.3	1.4	14.1	1.4
Middle distance, white	6	18.9	0.6	13.8	1.6
Middle distance, black	5	18.6	0.8	13.6	0.7
Distance, white	29	19.3	1.2	14.2	1.6
Jumps, white	9	19.3	0.9	15.1	1.8
Jumps, black	7	20.0	1.3	14.6	1.4
Throws, white	11	19.5	1.1	22.4	4.1
Throws, black	5	18.7	0.5	23.9	7.8

Relative fatness was estimated from predicted Db from the sum of four skinfolds skinfolds after Meleski et al [20]; see text.

Data from Malina RM, Battista RA, Siegel SR. Anthropometry of adult athletes: concepts, methods and applications. In: Driskell JA, Wolinsky I, editors. Nutritional assessment of athletes. Boca Raton (FL): CRC Press; 2002. p. 135–75.

hurdlers is only slightly lower than and overlaps the male reference, whereas corresponding estimates of % Fat in female athletes in these events are well below the female reference. (2) Percent Fat varies from early adolescence through adolescence into young adulthood in male and female middle distance and distance runners; it is considerably lower than the reference among female runners, whereas % Fat in male runners approximates the male reference at

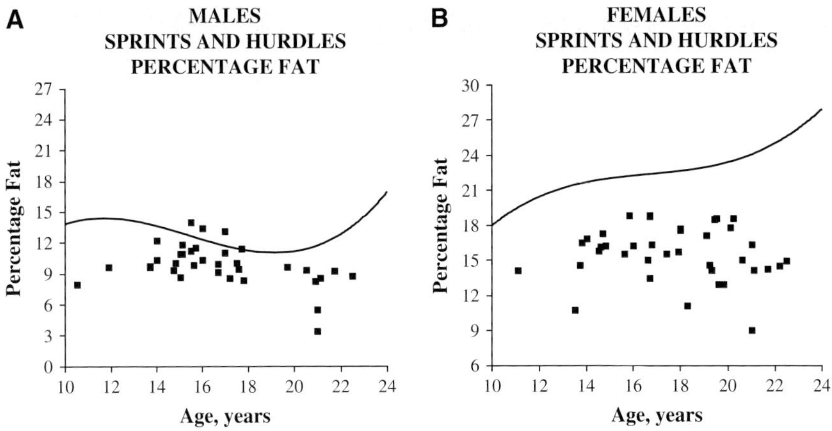

Fig. 2. Estimates of % Fat in samples of adolescent and young adult sprinters and hurdlers. (*A*) Males. (*B*) Females. (See ref. [50] for sources of data. Data for the nonathlete reference from Malina et al [35,39].)

many ages (3). The same general trend is apparent in jumpers and throwers. Percent Fat in female jumpers is well below the female reference, whereas it is quite close to the reference in male jumpers. Percent Fat in female throwers straddles the reference, but is above the reference in male throwers, especially in adolescence. Relative fatness tends to be lower in young adult compared with adolescent male throwers; such variation with age is lacking in female throwers.

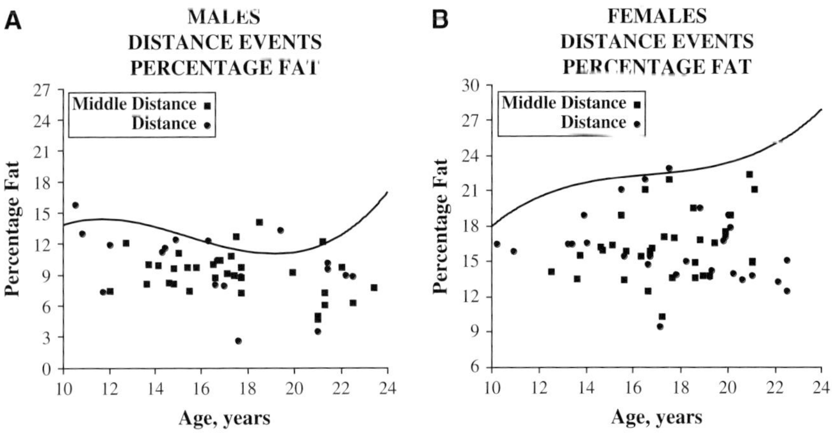

Fig. 3. Estimates of % Fat in samples of adolescent and young adult middle distance and distance runners. (*A*) Males. (*B*) Females. (See ref. [50] for sources of data. Data for the nonathlete reference from Malina et al [35,39].)

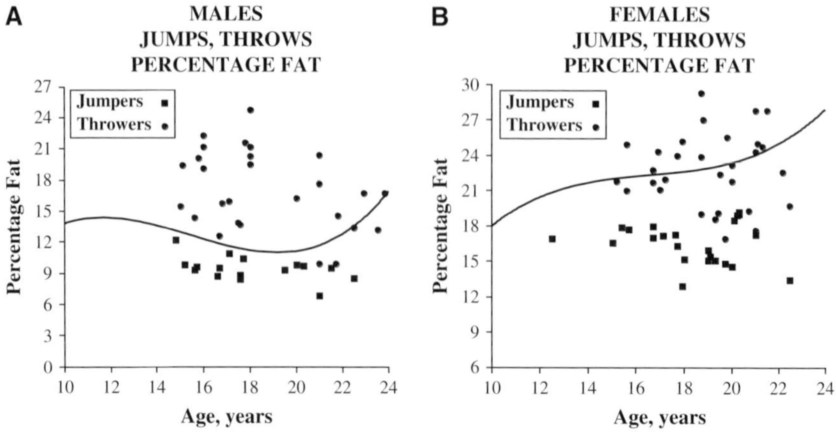

Fig. 4. Estimates of % Fat in samples of adolescent and young adult field athletes in jumping and throwing events. (*A*) Males. (*B*) Females. (See ref. [50] for sources of data. Data for the nonathlete reference from Malina et al [35,39].)

Wrestling

Weight management and specifically weight reduction are concerns in wrestling. Organizations associated with the sport have developed guidelines for minimum weight, defined as the lowest weight that an individual can maintain without comprising health [23]. Wrestling rules of the National Federation of State High School Associations [51] mandates the following:

> Each state association shall develop and use a weight-management program that includes a specific gravity not to exceed 1.025; a body fat assess no lower than seven percent for males/12 percent for females; and a monitored weekly weight loss plan not to exceed 1.5 percent a week.

The American College of Sports Medicine [52] suggests the following for young wrestlers:

> Assess the body composition of each wrestler before the season using valid methods for this population. Males 16 years old and younger with body fat below 7 percent or those over 16 with a body fat below 5 percent need medical clearance before being allowed to compete. Female wrestlers need minimal body fat of 12–14 percent.

The National Collegiate Athletic Association uses 5% Fat as the minimum allowable in weight certification formulas for wrestlers; however, body composition guidelines emphasize that estimates of body composition focus on a range of variation [53].

A key issue in putting the proposed guidelines into action relates to methods of estimating body composition and associated errors. Estimates derived from different methods may not be directly comparable. Some high school associations and school districts specify the type of estimate (DXA, BIA, skinfold measurements) at times with associated costs.

In one of the few detailed studies, body composition was assessed via hydrostatic weighing in the preseason, late season, and postseason in a sample of 9 male wrestlers 15.4 ± 0.3 years old [54,55]. Percent Fat at the three measuring points was 9.9 ± 0.5%, 8.0 ± 0.7% and 12.3 ± 0.8%. Corresponding estimates of FFM were 54.3 ± 3.1 kg, 53.2 ± 3 kg, and 56.2 ± 3.1 kg. The changes are relatively small and need to be viewed in the context of growth and maturation. Although body mass declined from the preseason to late season and increased into the postseason, linear growth, skeletal maturation, and growth-related hormones were not affected.

Among collegiate wrestlers competing at national tournaments (top 5–10% of wrestlers within each division), % Fat based on skinfold measurements was compared from the preseason to the competition [56]. Body mass and % Fat declined from the preseason to the tournament, 74.0 ± 11.1 kg to 71.5 ± 10.4 kg for mass and 12.3 ± 3.4% to 9.5 ± 1.8%. Mean minimal weights established for each wrestler in the preseason did not differ at the tournament.

TRAINING AND BODY COMPOSITION

Body composition is responsive to the demands of systematic training, as is evident in the observations on wrestlers. It is essential to consider separately observations in growing and maturing youth and in mature adults. Of relevance, are changes in body composition associated with training greater than those associated with normal growth and maturation? The increase in FFM (hydrostatic weighing) observed in youth regularly active in sport from 11 to 17 years old would seem to suggest an increase greater than that expected with normal growth and maturation [57,58]. This group of boys was larger in size and advanced in biologic maturation, however, compared with their age peers not engaged in sport. Similarly, among boys 11 to 13 years old undergoing a 5-month endurance training program, larger FFM (^{40}K) were observed in boys advanced in sexual maturation [59], suggesting perhaps that the boys were in their growth spurts [35]. The two studies highlight the difficulties in attempting to partition changes in body composition associated with training from 11 to 17 years old or with a short-term training program from the changes that accompany normal growth and maturation during male adolescence. Much of the variation in body composition in both studies was associated with a reduction in fatness.

Corresponding observations for girls are limited. A program of 30 minutes of high-impact aerobic and strength training activities three times per week for10 months was associated with increases in FFM (2.2 ± 1.1 kg) and FM (0.5 ± 0.8 kg) in 9- to 10-year-old girls [60]. Girls of the same age, body size, composition, and stage of sexual maturity who followed their normal pattern of activity for 10 months also increased in FFM (1.4 ± 1.4 kg) and FM (1.0 ± 0.8 kg). Both groups gained in FFM and FM, and there was, on average, no decrease in fatness. There also was considerable overlap between the trained and normal activity groups. Although the results are suggestive, they indicate difficulties inherent in attempting to partition growth-related from training-related changes in estimated body composition in adolescents [35].

Studies comparing changes in body composition associated with training in young adults generally compare pretraining and post-training means for FFM and % Fat, but duration of training programs and frequency of training vary. In addition, the samples do not comprise athletes. Using data reported by Wilmore [61], differences between pretraining and post-training means in nine studies of males 18 to 23 years old range from −0.2 kg to +1.4 kg for FFM (overall mean +0.8 kg) and −0.4% to −3.0% for relative fatness (overall mean −1.7%). Corresponding differences for 10 studies of females 18 to 22 years old range from −1.7 kg to +1.5 kg for FFM (overall mean +0.3 kg) and −2.1% to +3.1% for relative fatness (overall mean −0.4%). The persistence of changes associated with training are not usually considered; a relevant question is the following: How much training is needed to maintain changes in body composition induced by systematic training?

SEASONAL VARIATION IN BODY COMPOSITION IN ATHLETES

An issue related to the influence of training on body composition is changes in body composition of athletes during the course of a season. Studies commonly compare the body composition of athletes before and at the close of a competitive season [62,63]. Of potential relevance is variation in body composition associated with preseason or early season and in-season training protocols. This variation was considered in a sample of 15 elite university-level female swimmers who had their body composition estimated via densitometry at three points during a competitive season: October, December, and March [64]. Weight training with emphasis on high-repetition and low-resistance activities typically preceded swim training early in the season. Decreases in body mass (−1.3 ± 1.8 kg), FM (−2.4 ± 1.2 kg) and % Fat (−3.8 ± 1.9%) and an increase in FFM (1.1 ± 1.8 kg) characterized the early part of the season between October and December. These changes were generally maintained during the second part of the season, December to March, as the swimmers tapered in preparation for the national championships. Over this interval, changes in body mass (0.8 ± 1.2 kg), FM (0.8 ± 1.5 kg) and % Fat (1.2 ± 2%) were small, and FFM, on average, did not change (0 ± 1.1 kg). The results suggest that changes in body composition over the course of a season were concentrated primarily in the early part of the season. Corresponding changes in estimated body composition using anthropometric indicators have been described for female collegiate distance runners and basketball players [49].

BODY MASS INDEX AND ATHLETES

Many programs monitor the heights and weights of athletes in the form of the BMI. As noted, the BMI is reasonably well correlated with FM and % Fat in large and heterogeneous samples, but correlations between the BMI and FFM and FM are reasonably similar among youth [35]. A question of interest is the association between the BMI and indicators of body composition at the

Table 9
Correlations between the body mass index and estimates of fatness and muscularity in female university athletes and nonathletes grouped by category of body mass index

	Athletes							Nonathletes			
				Estimated Muscle Circumference						Estimated Muscle Circumference	
BMI (kg/m^2)				Arm		Calf				Arm	Calf
Category	*n*	∑8 skf	% Fat	T + B	T only	M + L	M only	*n*	% Fat	T only	M only
<18.5	14	0.68	0.64	0.10	−0.08	0.10	0.05	19	0.61	0.27	0.39
18.5 < 25.0	350	0.39	0.42	0.57	0.50	0.44	0.37	79	0.44	0.34	0.15
≥25.0	23	0.70	0.82	0.83	0.83	0.66	0.52	13	0.88	−0.36	−0.50

∑8 skf, sum of the triceps, biceps, forearm, subscapular, suprailiac, midthigh, medial calf, and lateral calf skinfold thicknesses; % Fat, based on predicted Db using an equation developed on elite female swimmers [20]; T+B, arm circumference corrected for the thickness of the triceps and biceps skinfolds; T only, arm circumference corrected for the thickness of the triceps skinfold only; M + L, calf circumference corrected for the thickness of the medial and lateral calf skinfolds; M only, calf circumference corrected for the thickness of the medial calf skinfold only [30].

Data from Malina RM, Battista RA, Siegel SR. Anthropometry of adult athletes concepts, methods and applications. In: Driskell JA, Wolinsky I, editors. Nutritional assessment of athletes. Boca Raton (FL): CRC Press; 2002. p. 135–75.

extremes of the BMI distribution. This was addressed in a large sample of female athletes using anthropometric indicators of body composition (Table 9). Although numbers of athletes with low (<18.5 kg/m^2) and high (≥ 25 kg/m^2) BMI are small, the trends in correlations suggest variable relationships. Among athletes with a BMI in the normal range ($18.5 < 25$ kg/m^2), correlations between estimates of fatness and muscularity are moderate and reasonably similar, ranging from 0.37 to 0.57. Correlations for % Fat and arm muscle are similar for nonathlete female college students with a BMI in the normal range, 0.44 and 0.34, although that for estimated calf muscle is lower, 0.15. Among those with a low BMI, correlations for fatness are higher and similar in athletes and nonathletes, 0.61 to 0.68. Correlations for estimated limb musculature and the BMI are low in athletes, -0.08 to 0.10, however, and higher in nonathletes, 0.27 and 0.39. Among those with a high BMI, correlations for fatness and estimated limb muscle circumferences are higher in athletes, 0.52 to 0.88, compared with athletes in the other two BMI categories. A similar high correlation, 0.88, is evident for % Fat in nonathletes with a high BMI, but correlations for limb musculature in nonathletes are negative. Overall, the data suggest variation in the association of the BMI and indirect estimates of fatness and muscularity at the extremes of the BMI distribution and indicate a need for further evaluation of the relationship between the BMI and body composition in athletes and nonathletes.

References

[1] Wang ZM, Pierson RN, Heymsfield SB. The five-level model: a new approach to organizing body composition research. Am J Clin Nutr 1992;56:19–28.

[2] Wang ZM, Shen W, Withers RT, et al. Multicomponent molecular-level models of body composition analysis. In: Heymsfield SB, Lohman TG, Wang ZM, editors. Human body composition. 2nd edition. Champaign (IL): Human Kinetics; 2005. p. 163–76.

[3] Roche AF, Heymsfield SB, Lohman TG, editors. Human body composition. Champaign (IL): Human Kinetics; 1996.

[4] Heymsfield SB, Lohman TG, Wang ZM, et al, editors. Human body composition. 2nd edition. Champaign (IL): Human Kinetics; 2005.

[5] Brozek J, Grande F, Anderson JT, et al. Densitometric analysis of body composition: revision of some quantitative assumptions. Ann N Y Acad Sci 1963;110:113–40.

[6] Siri WE. The gross composition of the body. Adv Biol Med Phys 1956;4:239–80.

[7] Going SB. Hydrodensitometry and air displacement plethysmography. In: Heymsfield SB, Lohman TG, Wang ZM, et al, editors. Human body composition. 2nd edition. Champaign (IL): Human Kinetics; 2005. p. 17–33.

[8] Schoeller DA. Hydrometry. In: Heymsfield SB, Lohman TG, Wang ZM, et al, editors. Human body composition. 2nd edition. Champaign (IL): Human Kinetics; 2005. p. 35–49.

[9] Ellis KJ. Whole-body counting and neutron activation analysis. In: Heymsfield SB, Lohman TG, Wang ZM, et al, editors. Human body composition. 2nd edition. Champaign (IL): Human Kinetics; 2005. p. 51–62.

[10] Forbes GB. Body composition in adolescence. In: Falkner F, Tanner JM, editors. Human growth, vol. 2. Postnatal growth, neurobiology. New York: Plenum; 1986. p. 119–45.

[11] Forbes GB. Human body composition: growth, aging, nutrition, and activity. New York: Springer-Verlag; 1987.

[12] Ellis KJ, Shypailo RJ, Abrams SA, et al. The reference child and adolescent models of body composition: a contemporary comparison. Ann N Y Acad Sci 2000;904:374–82.
[13] Malina RM. Variation in body composition associated with sex and ethnicity. In: Heymsfield SB, Lohman TG, Wang ZM, et al, editors. Human body composition. 2nd edition. Champaign (IL): Human Kinetics; 2005. p. 271–98.
[14] Lohman TG, Chen Z. Dual energy X-ray absorptiometry. In: Heymsfield SB, Lohman TG, Wang ZM, et al, editors. Human body composition. 2nd edition. Champaign (IL): Human Kinetics; 2005. p. 63–77.
[15] Goran MI. Energy expenditure, body composition, and disease risk in children and adolescents. Proc Nutr Soc 1997;56:195–209.
[16] National Institutes of Health. Bioelectrical impedance analysis in body composition measurement. Bethesda: NIH Technology Assessment Statement; 1994. p. 1–35.
[17] Chumlea WC, Sun SS. Bioelectrical impedance analysis. In: Heymsfield SB, Lohman TG, Wang ZM, et al, editors. Human body composition. 2nd edition. Champaign (IL): Human Kinetics; 2005. p. 79–88.
[18] Malina RM. Quantification of fat, muscle and bone in man. Clin Orthop 1969;65:9–38.
[19] Malina RM. The measurement of body composition. In: Johnston FE, Susanne C, Roche AF, editors. Human physical growth and maturation: methodologies and factors. New York: Plenum; 1980. p. 35–59.
[20] Meleski BW, Shoup RF, Malina RM. Size, physique and body composition of competitive female swimmers 11 through 20 years of age. Hum Biol 1982;54(3):609–25.
[21] Withers RT, Craig NP, Bourdon PC, et al. Relative body fat and anthropometric prediction of body density of male athletes. Eur J Appl Physiol 1987;56:191–200.
[22] Withers RT, Whittingham NO, Norton KI, et al. Relative body fat and anthropometric prediction of body density of female athletes. Eur J Appl Physiol 1987;56:169–80.
[23] Sinning WE. Body composition in athletes. In: Roche AF, Heymsfield SB, Lohman TG, editors. Human body composition. Champaign (IL): Human Kinetics; 1996. p. 257–73.
[24] Jackson AS, Pollock ML. Generalized equations for predicting body density of men. Br J Nutr 1978;40:497–504.
[25] Jackson AS, Pollock ML, Ward A. Generalized equations for predicting body density of women. Med Sci Sports Exerc 1980;12:175–82.
[26] Chumlea WC, Guo SS, Zeller CM, et al. Total body water reference values and predictions equations for adults. Kidney Int 2001;59:2250–8.
[27] Guo SS, Roche AF, Houtkooper LH. Fat-free mass in children and young adults from bioelectrical impedance and anthropometry variables. Am J Clin Nutr 1989;50: 435–43.
[28] Sun SS, Chumlea WC, Heymsfield SB, et al. Development of bioelectrical impedance analysis prediction equations for body composition with the use of a multicomponent model for use in epidemiological surveys. Am J Clin Nutr 2003;77:331–40.
[29] Warner ER, Fornetti WC, Jallo JJ, et al. A skinfold model to predict fat-free mass in female athletes. J Athl Train 2004;39:259–62.
[30] Malina RM. Anthropometry. In: Maud PJ, Foster C, editors. Physiological assessment of human fitness. Champaign (IL): Human Kinetics; 1995. p. 205–19.
[31] Sun SS, Chumlea WC. Statistical methods. In: Heymsfield SB, Lohman TG, Wang ZM, et al, editors. Human body composition. 2nd edition. Champaign (IL): Human Kinetics; 2005. p. 151–60.
[32] World Health Organization. Obesity: preventing and managing the global epidemic. Report of a WHO Consultation on Obesity. Geneva: WHO; 1998.
[33] Cole TJ, Bellizzi MC, Flegal KM, et al. Establishing a standard definition for child overweight and obesity worldwide: international survey. BMJ 2000;320:1240–3.
[34] Hedley AA, Ogden CL, Johnson CL, et al. Prevalence of overweight and obesity among US children, adolescents, and adults, 1999–2002. JAMA 2004;291:2847–50.

[35] Malina RM, Bouchard C, Bar-Or O. Growth, maturation, and physical activity. 2nd edition. Champaign (IL): Human Kinetics; 2004.
[36] Withers RT, LaForgia J, Heymsfield SB. Critical appraisal of the estimation of body composition via two-, three-, and four-compartment models. Am J Hum Biol 1999; 11:175–85.
[37] Moulton CR. Age and chemical development in mammals. J Biol Chem 1923;57: 79–97.
[38] Malina RM. Growth and maturation: normal variation and the effects of training. In: Gisolfi CV, Lamb DR, editors. Perspectives in exercise science and sports medicine, vol. II. Youth, exercise, and sport. Indianapolis: Benchmark Press; 1989. p. 223–65.
[39] Malina RM, Bouchard C, Beunen G. Human growth: selected aspects of current research on well nourished children. Ann Rev Anthropol 1988;17:187–219.
[40] Guo SS, Chumlea WC, Roche AF, et al. Age- and maturity-related changes in body composition during adolescence into adulthood: the Fels Longitudinal Study. Int J Obes 1997;21: 1167–75.
[41] Parizkova J. Growth and growth velocity of lean body mass and fat in adolescent boys. Pediatr Res 1976;10:647–50.
[42] Iuliano-Burns S, Mirwald RL, Bailey DA. The timing and magnitude of peak height velocity and peak tissue velocities for early, average and late maturing boys and girls. Am J Hum Biol 2001;13:1–8.
[43] Krawczyk B, Sklad M, Majle B. Body components of male and female athletes representing various sports. Biol Sport 1995;12:243–50.
[44] Schutte JE, Townsend EJ, Hugg J, et al. Density of lean body mass is greater in blacks than in whites. J Appl Physiol 1984;56:1647–9.
[45] Ortiz O, Russell M, Daley TL, et al. Differences in skeletal muscle and bone mineral mass between black and white females and their relevance to estimates of body composition. Am J Clin Nutr 1992;55:8–13.
[46] Gasperino JA, Wang J, Pierson RN, et al. Age-related changes in musculoskeletal mass between black and white women. Metabolism 1995;44:30–4.
[47] Gallagher D, Visser M, de Meersman RE, et al. Appendicular skeletal muscle mass: effects of age, gender, and ethnicity. J Appl Physiol 1997;83:229–39.
[48] Hortobagyi T, Israel RG, Houmard JA, et al. Comparison of four methods to assess body composition in black and white athletes. Int J Sport Nutr 1992;2:60–74.
[49] Malina RM, Battista RA, Siegel SR. Anthropometry of adult athletes: concepts, methods and applications. In: Driskell JA, Wolinsky I, editors. Nutritional assessment of athletes. Boca Raton (FL): CRC Press; 2002. p. 135–75.
[50] Malina RM. Crescita e maturazione di atleti bambini e adolescenti praticanti atletica leggera [Growth and maturation of child and adolescent track and field athletes]. Atletica Studi (Rome) 2006;(Suppl 1, 2):1–464.
[51] National Federation of State High School Assocations. 2006–07 wrestling rule changes. Available at: www.nfhs.org. Accessed July 10, 2006.
[52] American College of Sports Medicine. Current comment: weight loss in wrestlers. Indianapolis: American College of Sports Medicine; 1998.
[53] National Collegiate Athletic Association. 2006 NCAA Wrestling Rules and Interpretations, Appendix G. Assessment of body composition. Indianapolis: National Collegiate Athletic Association; 2005. Available at: http://www.ncaa.org/library/rules/2006/2006_wrestling_rules.pdf. Accessed July 10, 2006.
[54] Roemmich JN, Sinning WE. Weight loss and wrestling training: effects on nutrition, growth, maturation, body composition and strength. J Appl Physiol 1997;82: 1751–9.
[55] Roemmich JN, Sinning WE. Weight loss and wrestling training: effects on growth-related hormones. J Appl Physiol 1997;82:1760–4.

[56] Oppliger RA, Utter AC, Scott JR, et al. NCAA rule change improves weight loss among national championship wrestlers. Med Sci Sports Exerc 2006;38:963–70.
[57] Parizkova J. Longitudinal study of the relationship between body composition and anthropometric characteristics in boys during growth and development. Glasnik Antropoloskog Drustva Jugoslavije 1970;7:33–8.
[58] Parizkova J. Body fat and physical fitness. The Hague: Martinus Nijhoff; 1977.
[59] Von Dobeln W, Eriksson BO. Physical training, maximal oxygen uptake and dimensions of the oxygen transporting and metabolizing organs in boys 11–13 years of age. Acta Paediatr Scand 1972;61:653–60.
[60] Morris FL, Naughton GA, Gibbs JL, et al. Prospective ten-month exercise intervention in premenarcheal girls: positive effects on bone and lean mass. J Bone Min Res 1997;12: 1453–62.
[61] Wilmore JH. Appetite and body composition consequent to physical activity. Res Q 1983;54:415–25.
[62] Siders WA, Bolunchuk WW, Lukaski HC. Effects of participation in a collegiate sport season on body composition. J Sports Med Phys Fit 1991;31:571–6.
[63] Bolonchuk WW, Lukaski HC, Siders WA. The structural, functional, and nutritional adaptation of college basketball players over a season. J Sports Med Phys Fit 1991;31: 165–72.
[64] Meleski BW, Malina RM. Changes in body composition and physique of elite university-level female swimmers during a competitive season. J Sports Sci 1985;3:33–40.
[65] Fleck SJ. Body composition of elite American athletes. Am J Sports Med 1983;11: 398–403.
[66] Novak LP, Woodward WA, Bestit C, et al. Maximal aerobic power, body composition and anthropometry of Olympic runners and road cyclists. In: Jungmann H, editor. Sportwissenschaftliche Untersuchungen während der XX. Olympischen Spiele, München 1972. Hamburg: Karl Demeter; 1976. p. 79–90.
[67] Perez HR. The effects of competitive road-racing on the body composition, pulmonary function, and cardiovascular system of sport cyclists. J Sports Med Phys Fit 1981;21:165–72.
[68] Forbes GB. Toward a new dimension in human growth. Pediatrics 1965;36:825–35.
[69] Novak LP, Hyatt RE, Alexander JF. Body composition and physiologic function of athletes. JAMA 1968;205:764–70.
[70] Wickkiser JD, Kelly JM. The body composition of a college football team. Med Sci Sports 1975;7:199–202.
[71] Wilmore JH, Parr RB, Haskell WL, et al. Football pros' strengths—and CV weaknesses—charted. Phys Sportsmed 1976;4(Oct.):45–54.
[72] Novak LP, Bestit C, Mellerowicz H, et al. Maximal oxygen consumption, body composition and anthropometry of selected Olympic male athletes. In: Jungmann H, editor. Sportwissenschaftliche Untersuchungen während der XX. Olympischen Spiele, München 1972. Hamburg: Karl Demeter; 1976. p. 57–68.
[73] Raven PB, Gettman LR, Pollock ML, et al. A physiological evaluation of professional soccer players. Br J Sports Med 1976;10:209–16.
[74] Farmosi I, Apor P, Mecseki S, et al. Body composition of notable soccer players. Hung Rev Sports Med 1984;25:91–6.
[75] Agre JC, Casal DC, Leon AS, et al. Professional ice hockey players: physiologic, anthropometric and musculoskeletal characteristics. Arch Phys Med Rehab 1988;69:188–92.
[76] Sprynarova S, Parizkova J. Functional capacity and body composition in top weight lifters, swimmers, runners and skiers. Int Z Angew Physiol 1971;29:184–94.
[77] Sinning WE, Cunningham LN, Racaniello AP, et al. Body composition and somatotype of male and female Nordic skiers. Res Q 1977;48:741–9.
[78] Pollock ML, Pels AE, Foster C, et al. Comparison of male and female speed skating candidates. In: Landers DM, editor. Sports and elite performance. Champaign (IL): Human Kinetics; 1986. p. 143–52.

[79] Sinning WE, Wilson JR. Validity of generalized equations for body composition analysis in women athletes. Res Q Exerc Sport 1984;55:155–60.
[80] Fornetti WC, Pivarnik JM, Foley JM, et al. Reliability and validity of body composition measures in female athletes. J Appl Physiol 1999;87:1114–22.
[81] Novak LP, Woodward WA, Bestit C, et al. Working capacity (WC170), body composition, and anthropometry of Olympic female athletes. In: Jungmann H, editor. Sportwissenschaftliche Untersuchungen während der XX. Olympischen Spiele, München 1972. Hamburg: Karl Demeter; 1976. p. 69–78.
[82] Sinning WE. Anthropometric estimation of body density, fat, and lean body weight in women gymnasts. Med Sci Sports 1978;10:243–9.
[83] Colquhoun D, Chad KE. Physiological characteristics of Australian female soccer players after a competitive season. Aust J Sci Med Sport 1986;18:9–12.
[84] Fleck SJ, Case S, Puhl J, et al. Physical and physiological characteristics of elite women volleyball players. Can J Appl Sport Sci 1985;10:122–6.
[85] Piechaczek H. Oznaczanie tłuszczu ciała metodami densytometryczną i antropometryczna (estimation of body fat with densitometric and anthropometric methods). Mater Pr Antropol 1975;89:3–48.

Clin Sports Med 26 (2007) 69–89
CLINICS IN SPORTS MEDICINE

ELSEVIER
SAUNDERS

Female Athlete Triad Update

Katherine A. Beals, PhD, RD[a,*], Nanna L. Meyer, PhD, RD[a,b]

[a]Division of Nutrition, Department of Family and Preventive Medicine, University of Utah, Salt Lake City, UT 84112, USA
[b]The Orthopedic Specialty Hospital (TOSH Sport Science), 5848 South 280 East, Murray, UT 84107-6121, USA

The passage of Title IX legislation in 1972 provided enormous opportunities for women to reap the benefits of sports participation. For most female athletes, sports participation is a positive experience, providing improved physical fitness, enhanced self-esteem, and better physical and mental health [1]. Nonetheless, for a few female athletes, the desire for athletic success combined with the pressure to achieve a prescribed body weight may lead to the development of a triad of medical disorders including disordered eating, menstrual dysfunction, and low bone mineral density (BMD)–known collectively as the *female athlete triad* [1,2]. Alone or in combination, the disorders of the triad can have a negative impact on health and impair athletic performance.

HISTORY OF THE TRIAD

In 1992, a special American College of Sports Medicine (ACSM) Task Force on Women's Issues convened a consensus conference to discuss the incidence of three distinct, yet seemingly interrelated disorders–disordered eating, amenorrhea, and osteoporosis–seen in female athletes with increasing frequency. This combination of disorders was subsequently given the formal name of the *female athlete triad* (subsequently referred to in this article as the *triad*). Five years later, the ACSM published a position stand that not only documented the prevalence and consequences of the individual disorders of the triad, but also called for further research into the prevalence, causes, prevention, and treatment of the triad as a whole [2].

In the 9 years since the first Triad Position Stand was published, a significant amount of research has been completed. As a result, in 2003, the ACSM assembled a writing team of researchers and practitioners well versed in the area of the triad to develop a revised position stand, which is currently in its second set of reviews, but should be completed by the time this article is published. In addition to renaming the components of the triad, the new position stand

*Corresponding author. Division of Nutrition, Department of Family and Preventative Medicine, Salt Lake City, UT 84112. *E-mail address:* Katherine.Beals@hsc.utah.edu (K.A. Beals).

0278-5919/07/$ – see front matter
doi:10.1016/j.csm.2006.11.002
© 2007 Elsevier Inc. All rights reserved.
sportsmed.theclinics.com

proposes to emphasize many new concepts related to the triad, including the following [3]:

- New research related to the mechanisms involved in the pathogenesis of the triad disorders
- Low energy availability as the key disorder underlying the other components of the triad
- The spectrum that exists for each of the disorders—energy availability, menstrual function, and bone strength—ranging from health to disease as opposed to focusing only on the extreme end point of each disorder—clinical eating disorders, amenorrhea, and osteoporosis.

PREVALENCE OF THE TRIAD

Despite allegations that the triad is just a "myth" [4,5], and that researchers have grossly overestimated the extent of the problem [4–6], scientific data and anecdotal evidence indicate that the triad does exist and can have devastating consequences for female athletes [7–10]. Perhaps one of the reasons for the contradictory opinions regarding the magnitude of the problem stems from the dearth of solid data documenting the prevalence of the triad among female athletes. To date, only three studies have examined all three disorders of the triad using direct measures of BMD (ie, dual-energy x-ray absorptiometry [DXA]) in female athletes [7,10,11].

Beals and Hill [7] examined the prevalence of disordered eating, menstrual dysfunction, and low BMD among 112 US collegiate athletes representing seven different sports. Disordered eating and menstrual dysfunction were assessed by a validated health, weight, dieting, eating disorder, and menstrual history questionnaire, and BMD was determined via DXA. Although only one athlete met the criteria for all three disorders of the triad (using a Z-score ≤ -2.0), two additional athletes qualified when using a less conservative and more frequently used criterion for low BMD (ie, a Z-score < -1.0). In addition, 28 athletes met the criteria for disordered eating, 29 athletes met the criteria for menstrual dysfunction, and 2 athletes had low BMD (using a Z-score ≤ -2.0). Ten athletes met the criteria for two disorders of the triad using the more conservative BMD criterion, and this prevalence was increased to 13 athletes when the less conservative BMD criterion was used.

In a similar study, Nichols and colleagues [11] examined the prevalence of the triad of disorders among 170 high school athletes representing eight different sports. Disordered eating behaviors and attitudes were measured via the Eating Disorder Examination Questionnaire (Fairburn and Belgin, 1994), menstrual dysfunction was determined from a preparticipation examination questionnaire, and BMD was assessed via DXA (with a Z-score of ≤ -1 or ≤ -2 indicative of low BMD). Although only 2 athletes met the criteria for all three components of the triad, 10 girls met the criteria for two components; 18.2%, 23.5%, and 21.8% of the athletes met the criteria for disordered eating, menstrual dysfunction, and low BMD.

Using the entire population of elite Nowegian female athletes, Torstveit and Sundgot-Borgen [10] compared the prevalence of the triad among athletes with that of a nonathletic control group in a three-phase study design. In phase one, all athletes ($n = 930$) and all controls ($n = 900$) completed a detailed menstrual, weight, diet history, eating, and activity patterns questionnaire, which also included body dissatisfaction and drive for thinness subscales of the Eating Disorder Inventory (Garner et al, 1983). Based on data from phase one, a random sample of 300 athletes and 300 controls was selected and invited to complete a BMD test (phase two) and a clinical interview to ascertain eating disorder and disordered eating prevalence (phase three). A total of 186 athletes and 145 controls completed all three phases of the study, and of these, just 3 athletes and 3 controls presented with the full-blown triad. Compared with controls, a significantly greater percentage of athletes showed disordered eating and menstrual dysfunction (3.4% versus 10.8%; $P < .01$), whereas the opposite was found for menstrual dysfunction combined with low BMD (2.2% athletes versus 6.9% controls; $P < .05$).

These prevalence studies indicate that the number of athletes with all three disorders of the triad simultaneously is relatively small. Nonetheless, from a health and performance perspective, any occurrence, no matter how small, deserves attention. The percentage of athletes in all three studies with disordered eating and menstrual dysfunction was substantial and warrants concern. The finding that fewer female athletes have low BMD should not be surprising. First, as described in greater detail later, exercise, particularly that of a high-impact or bone-loading nature, has been shown to provide a protective effect on bone even under conditions of menstrual dysfunction or disordered eating [12–15]. Second, declines in BMD, particularly in the age groups of the female athletes routinely studied (ie, 13–25 years), can take a substantial amount of time to become apparent. Finally, research suggests that BMD may not be the best measure of bone "health," thus, currently available research may not accurately reflect the impact of disordered eating or menstrual dysfunction on bone health.

ETIOLOGY OF THE TRIAD

It is generally hypothesized that the development of the triad follows a typical progressive pattern. The female athlete, believing that a lower body weight would enhance athletic success, begins to diet. For numerous reasons, the athlete's diet becomes increasingly restrictive, her eating behaviors increasingly unhealthful. The resulting energy restriction and pathogenic weight control behaviors predispose her to menstrual dysfunction and subsequent decreased BMD [1,2]. According to this hypothesized scenario, the triad disorders are interrelated, such that the existence of one disorder is linked, directly or indirectly, to the others.

ENERGY AVAILABILITY

Spectrum of Energy Availability

As previously indicated, the revised ACSM Triad Position Stand will likely place a greater emphasis on the spectrum of behaviors and conditions within a given disorder category as opposed to the original version, which focused more on the extreme end point of each disorder category [3]. The category of *disordered eating* is meant to convey a continuum of abnormal eating behaviors, ranging from failing to meet the energy demands of exercise (ie, low energy availability) to the clinical eating disorders, anorexia nervosa, bulimia nervosa, and eating disorders not otherwise specified. Each one of the major categories contained within the spectrum of disordered eating is briefly described.

Clinical Eating Disorders

The clinical eating disorders include anorexia nervosa, bulimia nervosa, and eating disorders not otherwise specified (Table 1) [16]. To be diagnosed with a *clinical* eating disorder, an individual must meet a standard set of criteria outlined in the *Diagnostic and Statistical Manual of Mental Disorders,* 4th edition (DSM-IV) [16]. Clinical eating disorders are psychiatric conditions and go beyond simple body weight/shape dissatisfaction and involve more than just abnormal eating patterns or pathogenic weight control behaviors. Individuals with clinical eating disorders often display severe feelings of insecurity and worthlessness, have trouble identifying and displaying emotions, and experience difficulty forming close relationships with others [17]. In addition, clinical eating disorders are often accompanied by comorbid psychological conditions, such as obsessive-compulsive disorder, depression, and anxiety disorder [17].

Table 1
Clinical eating disorders

Anorexia nervosa
A significant loss of body weight, the maintenance of an extremely low body weight (85% of normal weight for height), or both
An intense fear of gaining weight or "becoming fat"
Severe body dissatisfaction and body image distortion
Amenorrhea (absence of $\geq$3 consecutive menstrual periods)
Bulimia nervosa
Episodes of binge eating (ie, consuming a large amount of food in a short period) followed by purging (via laxatives, diuretics, enemas, or self-induced vomiting) that have occurred at least twice a week for 3 mo
A sense of lack of control during the bingeing or purging episodes
Severe body image dissatisfaction and undue influence of body image on self-evaluation
Eating disorders not otherwise specified (EDNOS)
All the criteria for anorexia nervosa are met except amenorrhea
All the criteria for anorexia nervosa are met except that, despite significant weight loss, the individual's current weight is within the normal range
All the criteria for bulimia nervosa are met except that the binge and purge cycles occur at a frequency of less than twice a week for a duration of $<$3 mo
An individual of normal body weight regularly uses purging behaviors after eating small amounts of food (e.g., self-induced vomiting after consuming only 2 cookies)
An individual repeatedly chews and spits out, but does not swallow, large amounts of food

Adapted from American Psychological Association. Diagnostic and statistical manual of mental disorders. 4th edition. Washington, DC: APA; 1994.

Subclinical Eating Disorders

The term *subclinical eating disorder* is frequently used to describe individuals, athletes and nonathletes, who have considerable eating pathology and body weight concerns, but do not show significant psychopathology or fail to meet all of the DSM-IV criteria for anorexia nervosa, bulimia nervosa, or eating disorders not otherwise specified [18,19]. Many athletes who report using pathogenic weight control methods (eg, laxatives, diet pills, and excessive exercise) do not technically meet the criteria for a clinical eating disorder [19].

Low Energy Availability

Energy availability has been defined as the amount of dietary energy remaining for all other physiologic functions after energy has been expended in exercise [3]. Low energy availability results from consuming fewer calories than necessary to cover the additional energy demands of exercise. Although low energy availability can and often does result from disordered eating, it also can occur in the absence of disordered eating. An athlete unwittingly or unknowingly may fail to meet her exercise energy requirements because of time constraints, food availability issues, or lack of appropriate nutritional knowledge.

Prevalence of Low Energy Availability and Disordered Eating in Athletes

To date, no published studies have examined the prevalence of low energy availability among female athletes. Such research likely would prove difficult to conduct because it would necessitate accurately assessing energy intake and exercise energy expenditure. The limitations inherent in self-reported energy intake (eg, food records) and energy expenditure (eg, activity records) are well documented [20], and the expense or lack of generalizability involved in more direct measures (eg, metabolic feeding studies, doubly labeled water, whole room calorimetry) render such assessments impractical. Nonetheless, if it is assumed that most female athletes with disordered eating also are experiencing low energy availability, one can garner an estimate, albeit indirect, of prevalence.

Current estimates of the prevalence of disordered eating, including pathogenic weight control behaviors and subclinical and clinical eating disorders, range from less than 1% to 62% in female athletes [2,21,22] and 0% to 57% in male athletes [21,22]. These wide-ranging estimates are due to differences in screening instruments and assessment tools (eg, self-report questionnaires versus in-depth interviews), definitions of "eating disorders" employed (eg, few have used the DSM-IV criteria), and athletic populations studied (eg, collegiate versus high school athletes, elite athletes versus recreational athletes versus physically active people). Only four studies have used large ($N > 400$) heterogeneous samples of athletes and employed validated measures of disordered eating (Table 2) [23–26]. The remainder employed inadequate sample sizes, examined single sports, or used inappropriate measures of disordered eating, all of which can bias prevalence estimates.

Research suggests that the prevalence of disordered eating is higher in sports that emphasize a lean physique or a low body weight (ie, thin-build sports [23,25–27]). It has been hypothesized that the body weight demands of these

Table 2
Summary of prevalence studies including large, heterogeneous samples of athletes and validated assessments of disordered eating

Study	Subjects	Instrument	Findings
Beals and Manore (2002)	425 female collegiate athletes	EAT-26 and EDI-BD	3.3% and 2.4% of the athletes self-reported a diagnosis of clinical anorexia and bulimia nervosa; 15% and 31.5% of the athletes scored above the designated cutoff scores on the EAT-26 and EDI-BD
Johnson, Powers, and Dick (1999)	1445 collegiate athletes (883 men and 562 women) from 11 NCAA Division I Schools	EDI-2 and questionnaire developed by the authors using DSM-IV criteria	None of the men met the criteria for anorexia or bulimia nervosa; 1.1% of the women met the criteria for bulimia nervosa. 9.2% of the women and 0.01% of the men met the criteria for subclinical bulimia; 2.8% met the criteria for subclinical anorexia. 5.5% of the women and 2% of the men reported purging (vomiting, using laxatives or diuretics) on a weekly basis
Sundgot-Borgen (1993)	522 Norwegian elite female athletes	EDI and in-depth interview developed by the author based on DSM III criteria	1.3%, 8%, and 8.2% were diagnosed with anorexia nervosa, bulimia nervosa, and anorexia athletica
Sundgot-Borgen et al. (2004)	660 Norwegian elite female athletes	A 2-stage screening process including a questionnaire developed by the authors, including subscales of the EDI, weight history, and self-reported history of eating disorders (stage 1) followed by a clinical interview using the EDE (stage 2)	21% ($n = 21$) of the female athletes were classified "at risk" after the initial screening. Results of the clinical interview indicated that 2% met the criteria for anorexia nervosa, 6% for bulimia nervosa, 8% for eating disorders not otherwise specified (EDNOS) and 4% for anorexia athletica

Abbreviations: EAT-26, Eating Attitudes Test-26 [86]; EDI, Eating Disorder Inventory [87]; EDI-BD, Body dissatisfaction subscale of the EDI [87]; EDI-2, Eating Disorder Inventory 2 [88]; EDE, Eating Disorder Examination [89].

Data from Beals KA. Disordered eating among athletes: a comprehensive guide for health professionals. Champaign (IL): Human kinetics; 2004.

sports, and the pressure to achieve an ideal body weight, whether real or perceived, causes a female athlete to become overly concerned with her body weight and develop disordered eating behaviors [18,25].

Etiology of Disordered Eating in Athletes

Most eating disorder experts agree that there is no single "cause" of eating disorders among athletes, but rather that the etiology is multifactorial and encompasses a complex interaction between sociocultural, demographic, environmental, biologic, psychological, and behavioral factors [28]. Controversy currently exists whether athletes are at a greater risk for developing eating disorders than their nonathletic counterparts; some research suggests that the prevalence of disordered eating is greater among athletes [25,26,29], whereas other research does not [30,31]. The current controversy notwithstanding, evidence does suggest that certain inherent pressures in the sport setting may trigger the development of an eating disorder in psychologically vulnerable athletes.

Sundgot-Borgen [32] examined the etiology of disordered eating behaviors in 522 elite Norwegian female athletes and found that an early start of sport-specific training and dieting at an early age were frequently associated with the development of eating disorders. In addition, prolonged periods of dieting, frequent weight fluctuations, sudden increases in training volume, or traumatic life events (eg, an injury or a change of coach) tended to trigger the development of eating disorders.

Effects of Disordered Eating on Health and Performance

The effects of disordered eating on an athlete's performance vary, but largely depend on the severity and chronicity of the disordered eating behaviors and the physiologic demands of the sport [18]. An athlete who engages in severe energy restriction or who has been bingeing and purging for a long time is likely to experience a greater decrease in performance than one who has engaged in milder weight control behaviors for a shorter time. Likewise, athletes involved in endurance sports and other physical activities with high energy demands (eg, distance running, swimming, cycling, basketball, field hockey, and ice hockey) are likely to be more negatively affected than athletes involved in sports with lower energy demands (eg, diving, gymnastics, weightlifting). The potential consequences of disordered eating on health and performance are presented in Table 3.

MENSTRUAL DYSFUNCTION

Spectrum of Menstrual Function

The 1997 Triad Position Stand included only the extreme end point of menstrual dysfunction (ie, amenorrhea) [2]. The proposed revised triad uses the term *menstrual dysfunction* to depict more accurately the spectrum of menstrual irregularities that can plague female athletes, including luteal suppression (or shortened luteal phase), anovulation, oligomenorrhea, primary amenorrhea, and secondary amenorrhea [2,33]. In contrast to disordered eating and bone strength, menstrual irregularities do not exist on a continuum. An athlete

Table 3
Health performance consequences of disordered eating behaviors

Weight control behavior	Physiologic effects and health consequences
Fasting or starvation	Promotes loss of lean body mass, a decrease in metabolic rate, and a reduction in bone mineral density. Increases the risk of nutrient deficiencies. Promotes glycogen depletion, resulting in poor exercise performance
Diet pills	Typically function by suppressing appetite and may cause a slight increase in metabolic rate (if they contain ephedrine or caffeine). May induce rapid heart rate, anxiety, inability to concentrate, nervousness, inability to sleep, and dehydration. Any weight lost is quickly regained when use is discontinued
Diuretics	Weight loss is primarily water, and any weight lost is quickly regained when use is discontinued. Dehydration and electrolyte imbalances are common and may disrupt thermoregulatory function and induce cardiac arrhythmia
Laxatives or enemas	Weight loss is primarily water, and any weight lost is quickly regained when use is discontinued. Dehydration and electrolyte imbalances, constipation, cathartic colon (a condition in which the colon becomes unable to function properly on its own), and steatorrhea (excessive fat in the feces) are common. May be addictive, and athlete can develop resistance, requiring increasingly larger doses to produce the same effect (or even to induce a normal bowel movement)
Self-induced vomiting	Largely ineffective in promoting weight (body fat) loss. Large body water losses can lead to dehydration and electrolyte imbalances. Gastrointestinal problems, including esophagitis, esophageal perforation, and esophageal and stomach ulcers, are common. May promote erosion of tooth enamel and increase the risk for dental caries. Finger calluses and abrasions are often present
Fat-free diets	May be lacking in essential nutrients, especially fat-soluble vitamins and essential fatty acids. Total energy intake still must be reduced to produce weight loss. Many fat-free convenience foods are highly processed, with high sugar contents and few micronutrients unless the foods are fortified. The diet is often difficult to follow and may promote binge eating
Saunas	Weight loss is primarily water, and any weight lost is quickly regained when fluids are replaced. Dehydration and electrolyte imbalances are common and may disrupt thermoregulatory function and induce cardiac arrhythmia
Excessive exercise	Increases risk of staleness, chronic fatigue, illness, overuse injuries, and menstrual dysfunction

Data from Beals KA. Disordered eating among athletes: a comprehensive guide for health professionals. Champaign (IL): Human kinetics; 2004.

may or may not progress through subclinical menstrual disturbances before developing amenorrhea [34]. Conversely, an athlete may experience subclinical menstrual disturbances for years without ever experiencing a complete cessation of menstruation [34]. A brief description of the major categories of menstrual dysfunction is presented.

Luteal suppression
Also called luteal phase deficiency or shortened luteal phase, luteal suppression is generally an asymptomatic (ie, no overt symptoms) condition, characterized by a shortened luteal phase of the menstrual cycle (between ovulation and menstruation), which may be accompanied by a prolonged follicular phase (between menstruation and ovulation); the total cycle length remains relatively unchanged. Because there are no overt symptoms, luteal suppression can be diagnosed only by measuring ovarian steroid hormone concentrations in the blood or urine over an entire menstrual cycle [34]. Women with luteal suppression generally display low estradiol levels in the early follicular phase along with a slightly decreased luteinizing hormone (LH) pulse frequency and significantly increased pulse amplitude. The rate and extent of follicular development are reduced, ovulation occurs later, and the amount and duration of progesterone secretion during the luteal phase is reduced or shortened [34].

Anovulation
Anovulation is the absence of ovulation and is generally caused by impairment of follicular development resulting from altered hormonal status. More specifically, estrogen and progesterone levels are reduced; however, estrogen production is sufficient to stimulate some proliferation of the uterine lining, and bleeding often occurs. As a result, women with anovulation often do not realize that they are have a menstrual irregularity. In some instances, alterations in cycle length can occur, including very short cycles (<21 days) or overly long cycles (35–150 days) [34].

Oligomenorrhea
Literally translated, the term *oligomenorrhea* means "irregular menses." In practice, oligomenorrhea is used to describe a prolonged length of time between cycles (ie, >35 days) [33].

Amenorrhea
The term *amenorrhea* connotes the absence of menstruation and can be subdivided into two categories: primary and secondary. *Primary amenorrhea,* also referred to as *delayed menarche,* has been redefined by the American Society of Reproductive Medicine as the absence of menstruation by age 15 years in girls with secondary sex characteristics [35]. The age was lowered from 16 years due to the fact that age at menarche declined by 5 years in developed countries after the middle of the nineteenth century and is declining rapidly in developing countries. When amenorrhea occurs sometime after menarche, it is referred to as *secondary amenorrhea.* Generally, secondary amenorrhea requires the absence of at least three consecutive menstrual cycles [2].

Prevalence of Menstrual Dysfunction in Athletes
The prevalence of menstrual dysfunction among women in the general population who are not pregnant, lactating, or postmenopausal is estimated to be 2% to 5%, whereas the range is 6% to 79% among female athletes [2,36]. This wide

range of prevalence estimates seen in athletes can be largely explained by methodologic differences among the various studies that have attempted to measure menstrual dysfunction. Some of these methodologic issues are described.

- *Differences in the athletic population studied,* including the type of sport (ie, endurance versus esthetic versus strength/power; individual versus team sports), the level of competition (ie, elite versus recreational versus collegiate), and the age of the athlete. Small, nonrandomized studies that sample a single sport or athletes in similar types of sports may produce biased estimates of the incidence of menstrual dysfunction. For example, it is well known that menstrual dysfunction is common among distance runners [37–39]; if this population is used to represent the general female athlete population, it would likely produce an overestimation of prevalence. Conversely, if the sample is limited to female basketball or volleyball players (groups with a lower incidence of menstrual dysfunction), an underestimation of prevalence is likely to occur. To date, few studies have examined the range of menstrual disturbances in a large, heterogeneous group of female athletes.
- *Failure to control for oral contraceptive use.* Early prevalence studies in particular did not account for oral contraceptive use, or if they did, they did not indicate the rationale for use, which could confound prevalence estimates [34,40]. Many female athletes take oral contraceptives to regulate their menstrual cycle; if this is not taken into account, it could confound (ie, underestimate) the true prevalence of menstrual dysfunction.
- *Assessment of menstrual dysfunction.* Most prevalence studies have used self-report menstrual history questionnaires to ascertain menstrual dysfunction. Such questionnaires rely heavily on the honesty and accuracy of the individuals completing them and are subject to response bias. Even assuming honest responses, self-report may underestimate the incidence of menstrual dysfunction because many subclinical menstrual disturbances have no overt symptoms. Even studies that have attempted to verify self-report menstrual disturbances via measures of endocrine hormones generally investigated only a single menstrual cycle. Research by De Souza and colleagues [41] showed that data based on a single cycle grossly underestimate the actual incidence of menstrual disturbances.
- *Definitions of "menstrual dysfunction" used.* As previously indicated, researchers have used a variety of definitions for the different menstrual disturbances seen in athletes. which can have a great impact on the estimated prevalence. The more liberal the definitions used, the greater the prevalence. Johnson and associates [24] defined amenorrhea as one or fewer menstrual periods in 6 months and found that 6% of the athletes were amenorrheic. Fogelholm and Hiilloskorpii [27] reported that only 1% of athletes had amenorrhea, whereas the spectrum of menstrual dysfunction (including primary amenorrhea, secondary amenorrhea, and oligomenorrhea) among athletes not using oral contraceptives ranged from 32% to 37% (depending on the sport type examined—esthetic, speed, endurance, weight-dependent, or ballgame). These authors did not provide a clinical definition for the menstrual disturbances they examined; it is unclear what criteria were used for the various menstrual disturbances they examined. Beals and Manore [23] found that 31% of collegiate athletes studied reported *menstrual irregularity* (described

as cycles not occurring every 28–34 days), whereas 1% had no menstrual periods, 12% had fewer than 6 menstrual periods over the past year, and 8% had more than 12 menstrual periods over the past year. Dusek [38] found that 30% of a sample of 72 ballet dancers, runners, basketball players, and volleyball players experienced amenorrhea, defined as no menstruation for more than 3 months postmenarche. Finally, Torstveit and Sundgot-Borgen [42] reported that 31.4% of female athletes had menstrual dysfunction, which included primary amenorrhea (defined as absence of menarche by age 16 years), secondary amenorrhea (defined as an absence of three consecutive menstrual cycles), oligomenorrhea (defined by the authors as cycles of ≥35 days), and shortened luteal phase (defined by the authors as cycles of <22 days). These authors did not break the prevalence estimates down by menstrual dysfunction category.

Despite differences in the definitions used for menstrual dysfunction among the above-cited studies, without exception, all found that menstrual dysfunction was most evident among athletes participating in sports that emphasize leanness.

The estimated prevalence of delayed menarche among young women in the United States is less than 1% [9]. In contrast, Beals and Manore [23] found that 7.4% of a sample of 425 collegiate athletes (representing 15 different sports) reported not menstruating until after age 16 (as primary amenorrhea was previously defined), and 22.2% of athletes in esthetic sports (ie, cheerleading, diving, and gymnastics) reported primary amenorrhea.

The prevalence of oligomenorrhea also seems to be significantly higher among female athletes than the general female population [34]. Klentrou and Plyley [43] found that 61% of elite rhythmic gymnasts from Greece and Canada ($n = 45$) regularly experienced menstrual cycles longer than 35 days. Using a slightly different definition of oligomenorrhea (ie, more than three but fewer than nine cycles in 3 months), Burrows and coworkers [37] found the incidence among a group of English distance runners to be 21%. In a similar population (ie, English distance runners), Rosetta and colleagues [44] found a 40% total incidence of short (≤21 days) and long (≥35 days) cycles.

The lack of overt symptoms makes identifying luteal suppression or anovulation and consequently accurately assessing their prevalence among active women difficult. Nonetheless, both menstrual disorders are hypothesized to be common among female athletes. In regularly menstruating, recreational runners, the total incidence of luteal suppression and anovulation was 78% [34]. Similarly, Loucks and colleagues [45] found an 80% occurrence of luteal suppression in at least 1 of 3 consecutive months among a small group ($n = 9$) of "athletic" women.

Etiology of Menstrual Dysfunction in Athletes

Although the cessation of menses coincident with physical training has long been recognized, the specific etiology has yet to determined [2]. Endocrine and neuroendocrine experiments have shown that menstrual dysfunction in active women results from a disruption of the pulsatile secretion of LH by the pituitary gland–which is caused by a disruption of the pulsatile secretion of gonadotropin-releasing hormone by the hypothalamus. Nonetheless, the specific factor or factors responsible for these pulsatile disruptions remain largely unknown, although many possible theories have been proposed [36,45].

In the 1970s, low body weight or body fat was thought to be the primary cause of amenorrhea seen in physically active women [46,47]; however, subsequent research showed that a low body weight or body fat by itself cannot induce menstrual dysfunction [39]. Research indicates that neither body weight nor body composition varies significantly between amenorrheic and eumenorrheic athletes [39,48].

The so-called *exercise-stress* hypothesis purports that the stress of exercise training, similar to other chronic stressors, activates the hypothalamic-pituitary-adrenal axis, which disrupts the gonadotropin-releasing hormone pulse generator and results in menstrual dysfunction [9,36]. More recent research has shown, however, that it is not exercise per se that induces menstrual dysfunction, but rather an *energy deficit* [49–51]. This "energy deficit or energy drain" theory holds that failure to provide sufficient calories to meet energy requirements and support the carbohydrate needs of the brain causes an alteration in brain function that disrupts the gonadotropin-releasing hormone pulse generator through an as yet undetermined mechanism [49].

In a series of studies, Loucks and colleagues [49–51] showed that energy availability (or lack thereof) is at the root of hypothalamic menstrual dysfunction. In the first study, healthy, young, habitually sedentary, regularly menstruating women were subjected to four different experimental conditions designed to elicit energy balance and imbalance under exercise and calorie-restricted circumstances. In the exercise treatment groups, energy intake and energy expenditure (exercise) were controlled to set energy availability at an energy balance (approximately 45 kcal/kg lean body mass per day) and negative energy balance (approximately 10 kcal/kg lean body mass per day). In the nonexercising group, energy intake also was set to achieve energy balance and negative energy balance (to a similar degree as that for the exercising groups). The results indicated that exercise without a negative energy balance did not elicit significant disruptions in LH pulsatility. Low energy availability in the sedentary and exercising conditions produced marked alterations in LH pulsatility. The disruptive effects of low energy availability caused by exercise energy expenditure were smaller than those of dietary energy restriction [51].

In a follow-up study, it was determined that the "threshold" of energy availability (ie, the level of energy availability below which menstrual dysfunction is likely to occur) is approximately 30 kcal/kg lean body mass per day [49]. It was shown that the restoration of normal LH pulsatility in energetically disrupted women cannot be accomplished by a single day of aggressive refeeding, which provides further evidence for a mediating mechanism between energy availability and LH pulsatility.

Effects on Health and Performance

Female athletes who experience menstrual dysfunction, particularly amenorrhea, often show little concern for the disruption in their cycles; some even express relief at the "break." Similarly, some coaches simply dismiss menstrual dysfunction, believing it is a natural result of hard training [18]. Nonetheless, despite these attitudes, it should be emphasized that menstrual dysfunction is *not* a normal response to training; rather, it is a clear indication that health is being compromised. The health consequences of menstrual dysfunction are well documented and include infertility and other reproductive problems, decreased immune function, an increase in cardiovascular risk factors, and, perhaps most importantly, decreased BMD and increased risk for premature osteoporosis [2,52].

BONE HEALTH

Spectrum of Bone Health

The third component of the triad is related to the athlete's bone health. In the initial Triad Position Stand [2], this component was termed *osteoporosis,* which is defined as a degenerative skeletal disease most common to postmenopausal women and characterized by compromised bone strength [53]. Today, it is recognized that bone strength, as a triad component, also occurs along a spectrum that spans from low bone mass and stress fractures to osteoporosis, which is considered the most severe condition.

Bone strength not only is characterized by bone mineral content (BMC; g) and density (BMD; g/cm^2), but also by the quality of bone. The variation in bone strength is due to differences in BMC/BMD *and* bone quality [54]. Bone quality includes the microarchitecture or the three-dimensional array of trabeculae [55]. Bone quality refers to the process of bone turnover, or the dynamic nature of bone remodeling with osteoclasts breaking down bone (also known as bone resorption) and osteoblasts establishing a new matrix, or the osteoid, in the process of bone formation. Bone is a dynamic tissue that cycles over months. Osteoclasts mediate bone resorption via proteolytic digestion, followed by a delayed replacement of osteoclasts by osteoblasts, which lay down new bone or the matrix (osteoid). Until the matrix is fully mineralized, it takes several phases and hence time [56]. Finally, bone geometry and size also are important aspects of bone quality [57]. Differences in geometry and size are best explained by the gender difference in BMC and BMD, resulting mostly from a difference in cortical thickness between men and women who are of the same body size [58].

Although bone quality represents an important aspect of bone structure and strength, BMD assessed by DXA is currently the most accepted quantitative method for the diagnosis of osteoporosis and prediction of fracture risk [59]. It is likely that in the future, measures characterizing bone quality will be combined with BMD to describe the full scope of an individual's bone strength, as has been shown by Nikander and colleagues [60]. For the remainder of this article, however, the focus is on BMD measured by DXA, as it is currently used in the clinical setting to evaluate bone health and fracture risk in premenopausal and postmenopausal women [2,9,59,61].

Diagnosis of Low Bone Mass and Osteoporosis in Athletes

DXA has been used as a diagnostic tool for the evaluation of bone health and particularly low BMD. BMD is normally distributed and is often expressed in standard deviation (SD) units relative to its T or Z distribution. The T distribution has a mean of zero, which corresponds to the mean of young healthy women. T-scores are used for the diagnosis of osteoporosis and osteopenia and to predict fracture risk in postmenopausal women [59]. Specifically, the World Health Organization has established cutoff scores for the diagnosis of osteoporosis and osteopenia for postmenopausal women [59]. In postmenopausal women, fracture risk nearly doubles for every SD below the young adult mean [62]. One more recent debate has been related to the fact that the same diagnostic strategies used for postmenopausal women (the distribution of T-scores and the comparison with the young adult mean) have been applied to premenopausal women, adolescents, and children. This seems problematic for three reasons: (1) Fracture data are lacking in premenopausal women, (2) it can be assumed that fracture risk is low in young women, and (3) peak bone mass has not yet been attained in adolescents and children. The International Society for Clinical Densitometry (ISCD) currently is proposing that BMD comparisons in premenopausal women, adolescents, and children be made relative to chronologic age, using the Z distribution [61]. To avoid a disease label in premenopausal women and to account for a skeleton of a young woman around or younger than age 20 years that has not yet attained peak bone mass, the ISCD recommends using Z-scores. Z-scores are expressed relative to chronologic age and allow for a better comparison of BMD values in individuals younger than age 20 years. As women become older, however, Z and T distributions are similar. According to the ISCD 2005 Official Position [9], a young woman is no longer considered osteoporotic or osteopenic with a low Z-score or T-score. Instead, her BMD now is considered *low for chronologic age or is below the expected range for age*. Although the International Olympic Committee (IOC) (IOC Position Stand, 2005) is generally in agreement with the ISCD's approach, its diagnostic criteria seem more conservative when considering athletic women. This is probably due to the fact that athletes, in general, should have higher BMD than controls, as was previously discussed. For both organizations, the diagnosis of *osteoporosis* is still relevant, but should not be based on densitometric criteria alone and should integrate other factors, such as hypoestrogenism or eating disorders (see Table 4 for a summary) [9,61]. The aforementioned cutoff values are likely to change again, and an update of the Female Athlete Triad Position Stand through the ACSM is soon to be published as well.

In many instances and particularly in the athletic setting, DXA is not always available for the assessment and evaluation of an athlete's bone health. It is reasonable to assume, however, that an athlete's bone strength has suffered if she

Table 4
Current recommendations for the diagnosis of low bone mineral density and osteoporosis in premenopausal and postmenopausal women and young athletes

	World Health Organization	International Society of Clinical Densitometry	International Olympic Committee
Targeted population	Postmenopausal women	Premenopausal women	Young, premenopausal athletes
Terminology	Osteopenia	BMD below expected range for age	BMD below expected range for age
Proposed cutoff score	T-score: −1 to − 2.5	>20 years of age: Z-score*: ≤−2	>20 years of age: Z-or T-score: ≤−1 should be of concern
Terminology	Osteoporosis	Low BMD for chronologic age or below expected range for age	Osteoporosis in athlete with amenorrhea
Proposed cutoff score	T-score: ≤−2.5	<20 years of age: Z-score*: ≤−2	>20 years of age: Z-score*: −2.5

*Z-and T-score may be similar in young women >20 years old.
Data from references [9,59,61].

presents with amenorrhea for longer than 6 months or has experienced frequent phases of oligomenorrhea and possibly a stress fracture [9].

Prevalence of Low Bone Mass in Athletes

The prevalence of low bone mass and osteoporosis in athletes is difficult to address because of the differences in diagnostic criteria used among organizations and the fact that BMD data using DXA are not as easily and inexpensively collected. In general, using the World Health Organization classification for postmenopausal women [59], the prevalence of osteopenia in female athletes has been reported to be 22% to 50%, with a relatively low prevalence of osteoporosis [63]. Considering the new ISCD and IOC criteria, women with low T-scores or Z-scores would now be considered as having low BMD for chronologic age or below the expected range (ISCD Position Statement, 2005). More recently, Torstveit and Sundgot-Borgen [64] have applied these new criteria in a sample of 186 elite athletes and found that 10.7% had a BMD below the expected range for age.

Female athletes have higher BMD than their nonathletic counterparts. Athletes exhibit a BMD at several skeletal sites that is 5% to 15% higher than the BMD of nonathletes [65], even when controlled for confounding variables, such as age, body mass index, and lean body mass [64,66]. Sports with loading patterns that are characterized by high impact (basketball, volleyball, gymnastics) or odd impact (squash, speed skating, and other winter sports) are strongly associated with a higher BMD [60,64,66], whereas repetitive low-impact (running) [64] and non–weight bearing activities (swimming) are not [67].

It is not surprising that athletes, when healthy, have stronger bones than nonathletes. A study showed that low BMD is two to three times more common in controls compared with athletes [64]. Under the condition of menstrual dysfunction and the triad, however, this positive effect of exercise on bone is diminished.

When athletes have menstrual dysfunction, their BMD is significantly below that of their eumenorrheic counterparts [40,68,69], and in a sense, athletes lose the skeletal advantage of their sport involvement. Athletes with amenorrhea exhibit a BMD at the lumbar spine that is 10% to 20% below the BMD of eumenorrheic athletes [69,70]. Amenorrheic athletes also have significantly lower BMD at other skeletal sites compared with eumenorrheic athletes [71,72]. Oligomenorrhea and amenorrhea are detrimental to bone [73]; however, the impact of oligomenorrhea on BMD occurs likely at an intermediate stage along the spectrum of menstrual dysfunction [73,74]. Finally, the cumulative exposure of low estrogen in the form of oligomenorrhea or amenorrhea during an athlete's career also needs to be considered. The longer the duration of menstrual dysfunction, in the past and at present time, the lower the BMD [73].

Although most athletes with menstrual dysfunction present with lower BMD compared with their eumenorrheic counterparts, there are some exceptions. It has been shown that athletes in high-impact sports, despite menstrual dysfunction, seem to be able to maintain their higher BMD compared with athletes involved in lower impact sports who also have menstrual dysfunction [64] or eumenorrheic controls [75]. The mechanical loading patterns of certain sports may override the deleterious effect of hypoestrogenism.

Athletes with menstrual dysfunction are at greater risk not only for low BMD, but also stress fractures [23,66,72,76–78]. Torstveit and Sundgot-Borgen [78] identified that 17% of elite athletes reported having a stress fracture. Although not significantly different from normally active controls, the athletes were more likely to have menstrual dysfunction than the controls [78]. Besides stress fractures, athletes with one or more components of the triad also are more likely to report sprains, strains, and other soft tissue injuries [23], underlining the importance of the triad on health and the performance capabilities of young female athletes.

Etiology of Low Bone Mass in Athletes

The most important function of estrogen with respect to bone health is related to estrogen's suppressing effect on osteoclast activity [79]. As mentioned previously, osteoclasts are bone cells that tear down bone in the process of bone resorption. In the hypoestrogenic state, the female athlete likely exhibits accelerated bone resorption through the impact of irregular or absent menstrual cycles. In addition, a direct effect, through low energy availability, may be possible [80]. Some studies have shown that athletes, at risk for disordered eating, present with low BMD in the absence of menstrual dysfunction [74,78]. Studies aimed at correcting the hypoestrogenic state, using estradiol replacement (without an increase in energy intake), generally have not succeeded in the normalization of BMD after years of treatment [81–84], indicating that factors other than estrogen also are important for bone. The most convincing evidence that low energy availability may have a direct effect on bone was published in an article by Ihle and Loucks [85], who showed that markers of bone formation and resorption changed unfavorably within 5 days in sedentary women who were exposed to low energy availability through dietary restriction or increased exercise energy expenditure [85]. Whether this is also the case in athletic women has yet to be determined. Nevertheless, it seems highly plausible that an energy and nutrient deficit affects metabolic substrates and hormones, including insulin, growth hormone, insulin-like growth factor-1, cortisol, and thyroid hormone, which all are considered important hormones for bone metabolism, independent of the hypoestrogenic state [80].

SUMMARY

The 1997 ACSM Triad Position Stand concluded with a call for additional research regarding the prevalence, causes, consequences, prevention, and treatment of disordered eating, amenorrhea, and osteoporosis in female athletes. Almost a decade later, that call has been answered, and an updated version of the ACSM Triad Position Stand is pending. In addition to renaming the triad components to reflect the full spectrum of each–ranging from health to disease–the proposed revised version of the Triad Position Stand is expected to place a greater emphasis on low energy availability as the key disorder underlying the other components of the triad, include updated information regarding the prevalence of each component of the triad and the triad as a whole, and provide greater insight into the mechanisms involved in the pathogenesis of each disorder. Far from "setting health and social policies that ultimately discriminate against young women in the pursuit of athletic success" as more recent accusations have implied [5], advancing research and knowledge regarding the triad will aid in the creation of more efficacious prevention and treatment strategies so that all women can enjoy the physical, psychological, and social benefits of athletics participation to the fullest.

References

[1] Nattiv A, Agostini R, Drinkwater BL, et al. The female athlete triad: the inter-relatedness of disordered eating, amenorrhea, and osteoporosis. Clin Sports Med 1994;13(3):405–18.
[2] Otis CL, Drinkwater B, Johnson M, et al. American College of Sports Medicine position stand: the female athlete triad: disordered eating, amenorrhea, and osteoporosis. Med Sci Sports Exerc 1997;29(5):i–ix.
[3] The female athlete triad position stand—2004 update. Presented at MSSE 51st Annual meeting, Session E-40, Indianapolis (IN), June 2–5, 2004.
[4] DiPietro L, Stachenfeld NS. The myth of the female athlete triad. Br J Sports Med 2006; 40(6):490–3.
[5] DiPietro L, Stachenfeld NS, Pierce JB. The female athlete triad myth. Med Sci Sports Exerc 2006;38(4):795.

[6] Loucks AB. Methodological problems in studying the female athlete triad. Med Sci Sports Exerc 2006;38(5):1020.
[7] Beals KA, Hill AK. The prevalence of disordered eating, menstrual dysfunction, and low bone mineral density among US collegiate athletes. Int J Sport Nutr Exerc Metab 2006;16(1):1–23.
[8] Fredericson M, Kent K. Normalization of bone density in a previously amenorrheic runner with osteoporosis. Med Sci Sports Exerc 2005;37(9):1481–6.
[9] IOC Medical Commission Working Group Women in Sport. Position Stand on the Female Athlete Triad. Available at: www.olympic.org/common/asp/download_report. asp?file=en_report_917.pdf&id=917. Accessed June 1, 2006.
[10] Torstveit MK, Sundgot-Borgen J. The female athlete triad exists in both elite athletes and controls. Med Sci Sports Exerc 2005;37(9):1449–59.
[11] Nichols JF, Rauh MJ, Lawson MJ, et al. Prevalence of the female athlete triad syndrome among high school athletes. Arch Pediatr Adolesc Med 2006;160(2):137–42.
[12] Bemben DA, Buchanan TD, Bemben MG, et al. Influence of type of mechanical loading, menstrual status, and training season on bone density in young women athletes. J Strength Cond Res 2004;18(2):220–6.
[13] Laing EM, Wilson AR, Modlesky CM, et al. Initial years of recreational artistic gymnastics training improves lumbar spine bone mineral accrual in 4- to 8-year-old females. J Bone Miner Res 2005;20(3):509–19.
[14] Taaffe DR, Marcus R. The muscle strength and bone density relationship in young women: dependence on exercise status. J Sports Med Phys Fitness 2004;44:98–103.
[15] Taaffe DR, Robinson TL, Snow CM, et al. High-impact exercise promotes bone gain in well-trained female athletes. J Bone Miner Res 1997;12(2):255–60.
[16] American Psychological Association. Diagnostic and statistical manual of mental disorders. 4th edition. Washington, DC: APA; 1994.
[17] Fairburn CG, Brownell KD, editors. Eating disorders and obesity: a comprehensive handbook. 2nd edition. New York: Guilford Press; 2001.
[18] Beals KA. Disordered eating among athletes: a comprehensive guide for health professionals. Champaign (IL): Human Kinetics; 2004.
[19] Beals KA, Manore MM. Behavioral, psychological, and physical characteristics of female athletes with subclinical eating disorders. Int J Sport Nutr Exerc Metab 2000;10(2):128–43.
[20] Manore MM, Beals K. Dietary assessment. In: Dunford M, editor. Sports nutrition: a guide for the professional working with active people. 4th edition. Chicago: The American Dietetic Association; 2005. p. 145–59.
[21] Brownell KD, Rodin J. Prevalence of eating disorders in athletes. In: Brownell KD, Rodin J, Wilmore JH, editors. Eating, body weight and performance in athletes: disorders of modern society. Philadelphia: Lea & Febiger; 1992. p. 128–45.
[22] Byrne S, McLean N. Eating disorders in athletes: a review of the literature. J Sci Med Sport 2001;4(2):145–59.
[23] Beals KA, Manore MM. Disorders of the female athlete triad among collegiate athletes. Int J Sports Nutr Exerc Metab 2002;12(3):281–93.
[24] Johnson C, Powers PS, Dick RW. Athletes and eating disorders: the national collegiate athletic association study. Int J Eat Disord 1999;26(2):179–88.
[25] Sundgot-Borgen J. Prevalence of eating disorders in elite female athletes. Int J Sports Nutr 1993;3(1):29–40.
[26] Sundgot-Borgen J, Torstveit MK. Prevalence of eating disorders in elite athletes is higher than in the general population. Clin J Sport Med 2004;14(1):25–32.
[27] Fogelholm M, Hiilloskorpii H. Weight and diet concerns in Finnish female and male athletes. Med Sci Sports Exerc 1999;31(2):229–35.
[28] Brownell KD, Foryet JP, editors. Handbook of eating disorders: physiology, psychology, and treatment of obesity, anorexia nervosa, and bulimia nervosa. New York: Basic Books; 1986.

[29] Smolak L, Murnen SK, Ruble AE. Female athletes and eating problems: a meta-analysis. Int J Eat Disord 2000;27(4):371–80.

[30] Reinking MF, Alexander LE. Prevalence of disordered eating behaviors in undergraduate female collegiate athletes and nonathletes. J Athl Train 2005;40(1):47–51.

[31] Taub DE, Blinde EM. Eating disorders among adolescent female athletes: influence of athletic participation and sport team membership. Adolescence 1992;27(108): 833–48.

[32] Sundgot-Borgen J. Risk and trigger factors for the development of eating disorders in female athletes. Med Sci Sports Exerc 1994;26:414–9.

[33] Otis CL. Exercise-associated amenorrhea. Clin Sports Med 1992;11(2):351–62.

[34] Redman LM, Loucks AB. Menstrual disorders in athletes. Sports Med 2005;35(9):747–55.

[35] Practice Committee of the American Society for Reproductive Medicine. Current evaluation of amenorrhea. Fertil Steril 2004;82:266–72.

[36] Warren MP, Perlroth NE. The effects of intense exercise on the female reproductive system. J Endocrinol 2001;170:3–11.

[37] Burrows M, Nevill AM, Bird S, et al. Physiological factors associated with low bone mineral density in female endurance runners. Br J Sports Med 2003;37(1):67–71.

[38] Dusek T. Influence of high intensity training on menstrual cycle disorders in athletes. Croat Med J 2001;42:79–82.

[39] Sanborn CF, Albrecht BH, Wagner WW. Athletic amenorrhea: lack of association with body fat. Med Sci Sports Exerc 1987;19(3):207–12.

[40] Marcus R, Cann C, Madvig P, et al. Menstrual function and bone mass in elite women distance runners: endocrine and metabolic features. Ann Intern Med 1985;102(2): 158–63.

[41] De Souza MJ, Molle BE, Loucks AB, et al. High frequency of luteal phase deficiency and anovulation in recreational women runners, blunted elevation in follicular stimulatings hormones observed during luteal follicular transition. J Clin Endocrinol Metab 1998;83(12): 4220–32.

[42] Torstveit MK, Sundgot-Borgen J. Participation in leanness sports but not training volume is associated with menstrual dysfunction: a national survey of 1,276 elite athletes and controls. Br J Sports Med 2005;39(3):141–7.

[43] Klentrou P, Plyley M. Onset of puberty, menstrual frequency, and body fat in elite rhythmic gymnasts compared with normal controls. Br J Sports Med 2003;37(6):490–4.

[44] Rosetta L, Harrison GA, Read GF. Ovarian impairments of female recreational distance runners. Ann Hum Biol 1998;25(4):345–57.

[45] Loucks AB, Mortola JF, Girton L, et al. Alterations in the hypothalamic-pituitary-ovarian and the hypothalamic-pituitary-adrenal axes in athletic women. J Clin Endocrinol Metab 1989; 68(2):402–11.

[46] Frisch RE, McArthur JW. Menstrual cycles: fatness as a determinant of minimum weight for height necessary for their maintenance or onset. Science 1974;185(4155):949–51.

[47] Frisch RE, Revelle R. Height and weight at menarche and a hypothesis of menarche. Arch Dis Child 1971;46(2):695–701.

[48] Loucks AB, Horvath SM. Exercise-induced stress responses of amenorrheic and eumenorrheic runners. J Clin Endocrinol Metab 1984;59(6):1109–20.

[49] Loucks AB, Thuma JR. Luteinizing hormone pulsatility is disrupted at a threshold of energy availability in regularly menstruating women. J Clin Endocrinol Metab 2003;88(1): 297–311.

[50] Loucks AB, Verdun M. Slow restoration of LH pulsatility by refeeding in energetically disrupted women. Am J Physiol 1998;275:R1218–26.

[51] Loucks AB, Verdun M, Heath EM. Low energy availability, not stress of exercise, alters LH pulsatility in exercising women. J Appl Physiol 1998;84(1):37–46.

[52] Constantini NA. Clinical consequences of athletic amenorrhea. Sports Med 1994;17(4): 213–23.

[53] National Institutes of Health. Osteoporosis prevention, diagnosis, and therapy. NIH Consens Statement 2000;17(1):1–45.
[54] Rubin CD. Emerging concepts in osteoporosis and bone strength. Curr Med Res Opin 2005;21(7):1049–56.
[55] Dalle Carbonare L, Giannini S. Bone microarchitecture as an important determinant of bone strength. J Endocrinol Invest 2004;27(7–8):99–105.
[56] Holick MF. Introduction to bone and mineral metabolism: bone structure and metabolism. In: Braunwald EF, Kasper AS, Hauser DL, et al, editors. Harrison's principles of internal medicine. New York: McGraw-Hill; 2001. p. 2192–205.
[57] Turner CH. Biomechanics of bone: determinants of skeletal fragility and bone quality. Osteoporos Int 2002;13(2):97–104.
[58] Nieves JW, Formica C, Ruffing J, et al. Males have larger skeletal size and bone mass than females, despite comparable body size. J Bone Miner Res 2005;20(3):529–35.
[59] World Health Organization. Assessment of fracture risk and its application to screening for postmenopausal osteoporosis. Geneva: WHO; 1994.
[60] Nikander R, Sievanen H, Heinonen A, et al. Femoral neck structure in adult female athletes subjected to different loading modalities. J Bone Miner Res 2005;20(3):520–8.
[61] Leib ES, Lewiecki EM, Binkley N, et al. Official positions of the international society for clinical densitometry. J Clin Densitometry 2004;7(1):1–6.
[62] Marshall D, Johnell O, Wedel H. Meta-analysis of how well measures of bone mineral density predict occurrence of osteoporotic fractures. BMJ 1996;312(7041):1254–9.
[63] Kahn KM, Liu-Ambrose T, Sran MM, et al. New criteria for the female athlete triad. Br J Sports Med 2002;36:10–3.
[64] Torstveit MK, Sundgot-Borgen J. Low bone mineral density is two to three times more prevalent in non-athletic premenopausal women than in elite athletes: a comprehensive controlled study. Br J Sports Med 2005;39(5):282–7 [discussion 282–7].
[65] Nichols DL, Bonnick SL, Sanborn CF. Bone health and osteoporosis. Clin Sports Med 2004;19(2):233–49.
[66] Meyer NL, Shaw JM, Manore MM, et al. Bone mineral density of Olympic-level female winter sport athletes. Med Sci Sports Exec 2004;36(9):1594–601.
[67] Taaffe DR, Snow-Harter C, Connolly DA, et al. Differential effects of swimming versus weight-bearing activity on bone mineral status of eumenorrheic athletes. J Bone Miner Res 1995;10(4):586–93.
[68] Cann CE, Martin MC, Genant HK, et al. Decreased spinal mineral content in amenorrheic women. JAMA 1984;251(5):626–9.
[69] Drinkwater BL, Nilson K, Chesnut CH III, et al. Bone mineral content of amenorrheic and eumenorrheic athletes. N Engl J Med 1984;311(5):277–81.
[70] Bennell KL, Malcolm SA, Ward JD, et al. Skeletal effects of menstrual disturbances in athletes. Scand J Med Sci Sports 1997;7:261–73.
[71] Myburgh KH, Bachrach LK, Lewis B, et al. Low bone mineral density at axial and appendicular sites in amenorrheic athletes. Med Sci Sports Exerc 1993;25(11):1197–202.
[72] Rencken ML, Chesnut CH III, Drinkwater BL. Bone density at multiple skeletal sites in amenorrheic athletes. JAMA 1996;276(3):238–40.
[73] Drinkwater BL, Bruemner B, Chesnut CH III. Menstrual history as a determinant of current bone density in young athletes. JAMA 1990;263(4):545–8.
[74] Cobb KL, Bachrach LK, Greendale G, et al. Disordered eating, menstrual irregularity, and bone mineral density in female runners. Med Sci Sports Exerc 2003;35(5):711–9.
[75] Robinson TL, Snow-Harter C, Taaffe DR, et al. Gymnasts exhibit higher bone mass than runners despite similar prevalence of amenorrhea and oligomenorrhea. J Bone Miner Res 1995;10(1):26–35.
[76] Carbon RJ. Exercise, amenorrhoea and the skeleton. Br Med Bull 1992;48(3):546–60.
[77] Eller DJ, Katz DS, Bergman AG, et al. Sacral stress fractures in long-distance runners. Clin J Sport Med 1997;7(3):222–5.

[78] Torstveit MK, Sundgot-Borgen J. The female athlete triad: are elite athletes at increased risk? Med Sci Sports Exerc 2005;37(9):184–93.

[79] Riggs BL, Khosla S, Atkinson EJ, et al. Evidence that type I osteoporosis results from enhanced responsiveness of bone to estrogen deficiency. Osteoporos Int 2003;14(9): 728–33.

[80] De Souza MJ, Williams NI. Beyond hypoestrogenism in amenorrheic athletes: energy deficiency as a contributing factor for bone loss. Curr Sports Med Rep 2005;4(1):38–44.

[81] Drinkwater BL, Nilson K, Ott S, et al. Bone mineral density after resumption of menses in amenorrheic athletes. JAMA 1986;256(3):380–2.

[82] Haenggi W, Casez JP, Birkhaeuser MH, et al. Bone mineral density in young women with long-standing amenorrhea: limited effect of hormone replacement therapy with ethinylestradiol and desogestrel. Osteoporos Int 1984;4(2):99–103.

[83] Keen AD, Drinkwater BL. Irreversible bone loss in former amenorrheic athletes. Osteoporos Int 1997;7(4):311–5.

[84] Warren MP, Brooks-Gunn J, Fox RP, et al. Persistent osteopenia in ballet dancers with amenorrhea and delayed menarche despite hormone therapy: a longitudinal study. Fertil Steril 2003;80(2):398–404.

[85] Ihle R, Loucks AB. Dose-response relationships between energy availability and bone turnover in young exercising women. J Bone Miner Res 2004;19(8):1231–40.

[86] Garner DM, Olmstead MP, Bohr Y, et al. The Eating Attitudes Test: psychometric features and clinical correlates. Psychol Med 1982;12(4):871–8.

[87] Garner DM, Olmstead MP, Polivy P. Development and validation of a multidimensional Eating Disorder Inventory for anorexia nervosa and bulimia. Int J Eat Disord 1983;2:15–34.

[88] Garner DM. Eating Disorder Inventory–2 manual. Odessa (FL): Psychological Assessment Resources; 1991.

[89] Cooper Z, Cooper PJ, Fairburn CG. The validity of the eating disorder examination and its subscales. Br J Psychiatry 1989;154:807–12.

Clin Sports Med 26 (2007) 91–100
CLINICS IN SPORTS MEDICINE

ELSEVIER SAUNDERS

Nutrition Recommendations for Masters Athletes

Christine A. Rosenbloom, PhD, RD*, Ann Dunaway
Division of Nutrition, Georgia State University, 140 Decatur Street, Suite 816, Georgia State University, Atlanta, GA 30303, USA

"More than 3000 masters athletes from 62 countries compete in Linz, Austria, in March of 2006" [1]. In 2005, 9000 "silver-haired Americans go for the gold" [2]. The National Senior Games Association announced a "major change in the NSGA rules affecting the game of basketball; a new age division of 80+ has been added for 2007" [3].

The above-mentioned athletes are competing at the masters level. Masters athletes are defined differently by every organizational body, but for purposes of this article, masters athletes are athletes older than 50 years old.

Even professional athletes are pushing the idea that sports are not only for young participants. The National Football League reported that 43 players have played until the age of 40. In the 2005 season, 9 players older than 40 were active, including a 45-year-old kicker for the Tennessee Titans [4].

The news that athletes are competing at older ages should not be a surprise when one considers the aging of the US population. In 2006, the oldest of the baby boomers turned 60 [5]. The Administration on Aging estimates that 7918 people will turn 60 every day, or about 330 every hour [5]. Although exact numbers are unavailable, it is accurate to say that today's generation of older adults is more active than their parents or grandparents. Twenty-three percent of health club memberships in the United States belong to adults older than age 55 [6]. Consider the increase in participation in the Huntsman World Senior Games held annually in Utah. This competition is open to all athletes age 50 or older. In 1987, 500 participants competed in a variety of sports; in 2005, 9000 athletes from around the world competed in basketball, tennis, cycling, mountain biking, racquetball, road racing, swimming, triathlon, track and field, volleyball, and softball [2].

HEALTH BENEFITS OF ATHLETIC PARTICIPATION

The literature on the health benefits of participating in masters athletics indicates that these athletes have favorable lipid profiles, normal insulin and glucose levels with no age-related deterioration of glucose tolerance, good bone

*Corresponding author. *E-mail address*: crosenboom@gsu.edu (C.A. Rosenbloom).

0278-5919/07/$ – see front matter
doi:10.1016/j.csm.2006.11.005

© 2007 Elsevier Inc. All rights reserved.
sportsmed.theclinics.com

health, and improved mood states compared with age-matched sedentary controls [7–10]. More extensive reviews on the physiologic and psychological benefits of participating in vigorous activity at the masters level of competition have been published [11,12], but one thing is clear: The benefits to health continue as long as the older athlete is active. When activity ceases because of injury or disinterest, the health benefits recede.

RESTING METABOLIC RATE AND CHANGES IN BODY COMPOSITION

Aging brings on alterations in resting metabolic rate (RMR) and changes in body composition. Aging is associated with declines in all components of energy expenditure: RMR, thermic effect of food, and energy expenditure [13]. Early research suggested an inverse relationship between RMR and aging (the older one got, the more decline in RMR was seen), but more recent studies suggest that the age-related decline in RMR can be attenuated by regular exercise [14]. Van Pelt and colleagues [15,16] studied RMR in men and women. Sixty-five healthy women (21–35 years old and 50–72 years old) were recruited to study age-related decline in RMR. Subjects were divided into groups of controls, endurance-trained runners, or swimmers. The primary finding from the study is that the decline expected in RMR with aging is attenuated in older women who remain physically active [15]. The research group conducted a similar study with men ($n = 137$; 19–36 years old and 52–75 years old). They reported that adjusted RMR declines with age even in physically active men, but the decrease in RMR is related to reductions in training volume and energy intake, which contribute to altered body composition. In the group of older men who maintained a high level of training and adequate energy intake, there was no significant difference in RMR compared with the younger age groups [16].

These data are applicable to masters athletes and may provide motivation for continued participation in sports. Women in particular are concerned with weight gain after menopause. Postmenopausal women have higher body fat levels and more central obesity than premenopausal women, but several investigations reveal that lifestyle, especially physical activity, is more responsible for alterations in body composition than hormone status [17]. Data from the Third National Health and Nutrition Examination Survey also indicated that women age 25 to 55 who met or exceeded the exercise guidelines to be moderately active 5 days a week or vigorously active for 3 days a week had lower body mass index, percent body fat, and waist-to-hip ratios than less active women [18].

NUTRITION RECOMMENDATIONS

Energy Intake

There are few published data on the energy needs of masters athletes; the key factor for predicting energy needs in masters athletes is training volume. The Dietary Reference Intakes (DRIs) for energy and macronutrient intakes can be used as a guide in establishing energy requirements [19]. The DRIs set estimated energy requirements for four different levels of exercise. Using the "active" physical activity level, Table 1 shows estimated energy requirements for older adults. These levels should be used only as a guide; competitive masters athletes with heavy training loads could require more calories to fuel training and activity.

Carbohydrate

The DRIs suggest dietary carbohydrate should be in the range of 45% to 65% of total calories [18]. For athletes, calculating carbohydrate needs based on grams per kilogram of body weight is more likely to meet the athlete's need for fuel. Consider an older female athlete who weighs 120 lb and has an estimated energy need of 2116 calories. Forty-five percent of energy from carbohydrate would yield 238 g of carbohydrate for daily needs. Using the recommendations of 5 to 7 g/kg/d for general training needs, this woman would need 272 to 380 g of carbohydrate. The typical US diet provides 4 to 5 g/kg/d, and athletes who train daily and compete at high intensity need more carbohydrate [20]. Endurance athletes require 7 to 10 g/kg/d, and athletes participating in ultraendurance events need more than 10 g/kg/d.

Carbohydrate feedings during exercise that lasts more than 1 hour can improve performance and help athletes have a "kick" at the end of a sprint [20]. It is recommended that 30 to 60 g of carbohydrate (in food or beverage) be consumed every hour. This is not a large volume of food, and athletes should be encouraged to experiment during training with foods that are portable, easy to eat, and do not cause gastrointestinal upset. Energy bars are often eaten because of their convenience, and perhaps because of their persuasive marketing to athletes, but there is nothing magical about energy bars. Fig Newtons, dried fruit, or crackers also can provide needed carbohydrate.

Recovery from hard exercise (>90 minutes) is enhanced with a carbohydrate feeding in the immediate postexercise period [20]. Athletes should aim to get 1.5 g/kg immediately after exercise if they are training daily. An additional carbohydrate feeding 2 hours later enhances muscle glycogen synthesis. These recommendations are for athletes who train hard and train daily; a 5-km road racer who competes once a month does not need to worry about recovery carbohydrate.

Table 1
Estimated energy requirements for older adults who are active

Age group in years	Men (kcal/d)	Women (kcal/d)
50–59	2757	2186
60–69	2657	2116
70–70	2557	2046
80–89	2457	1967

Data from Institute of Medicine. Dietary reference intakes for energy, carbohydrates, fiber, fat, protein and amino acids (macronutrients). Washington, DC: National Academy Press; 2002. Available at: http://www.nap.edu/books. Accessed March 30, 2006.

Protein

Usual aging is associated with declines in lean muscle mass. The term *sarcopenia* has been coined to describe the decline in skeletal muscle mass and concomitant loss of muscle strength with aging [21,22]. The prevalence of sarcopenia may be 30% for adults older than age 60 years, and it can lead to reduced function and disability for older men and women [22]. Physical activity, especially progressive resistance training, may be the best antidote to sarcopenia. Nutritional strategies also are being studied to assess the appropriate level of protein and amino acids in the diet.

Protein recommendations for masters athletes have not been established, but it is suggested that the same guidelines for younger athletes are appropriate. Protein in the range of 1.2 to 1.7 g/kg/d should provide adequate supplies of amino acids for muscle synthesis and repair. There is debate over the adequacy of the current Recommended Dietary Allowance (RDA) for protein for older adults. Several studies suggest that the current RDA of 0.8 g/kg/d is insufficient for maintaining positive nitrogen balance or providing sufficient anabolic stimulus for muscle repair [23,24].

Two considerations for protein intake for masters athletes are warranted. The first is adequate energy intake; the body's primary need is for energy, and protein can be converted to glucose if the body needs fuel. Assessing energy and protein needs in masters athletes is important to ensure that protein is used for anabolic functions and not for energy needs. Second, the timing of protein intake may influence the anabolic stimulus for muscle repair and growth. Ingestion of small amounts of protein (0.1–0.2 g/kg/h) can enhance muscle anabolism during recovery from endurance and resistance exercise [25]. To date, research studies showing this effect have used essential amino acids. Recommending that masters athletes consume small snacks of foods that provide essential amino acids may enhance muscle building and recovery. Foods and fluids that meet these criteria include milk, eggs, cheese, yogurt, lean meat, fish, and poultry.

Fat

The DRIs recommend a range of fat intake of 20% to 35% of total calories [19]. Heart healthy fats (monounsaturated and long-chain polyunsaturated fats) are recommended to provide essential fatty acids and improve blood lipids levels. No recommendation for dietary fat is available for masters athletes, and the American Dietetic Association recommends that athletes not restrict their fat intake because no benefit to performance with a low-fat diet has been identified [26].

Micronutrients

There has been little research to date on the micronutrient needs of masters athletes. Although there is evidence of benefit to altering the micronutrient needs of older adults in the general population, there are few guidelines for older adults who are physically active, much less engage in regular, strenuous exercise. For adults older than 50 years, the DRIs have established increased needs for vitamin D, calcium, and vitamin B_6. Other nutrients of interest for older adults are folate and vitamin B_{12}. For women older than 50 years, the iron requirement is decreased to the same level needed for men. Limited research exists for thiamine, riboflavin, choline, and zinc.

Vitamin D

In a study of 18 French male masters athletes with a mean age of 63 years, it was found that despite an increased energy intake compared with the French recommended dietary allowance, the men were deficient in vitamin D intake [27]. The average intake was 2.1 μg/d, which is far below the recommended levels. Older adults have higher requirements of vitamin D because the skin is less able to synthesize vitamin D from the sun. In addition, there is less 25-hydroxyvitamin D circulating in the blood with advancing age. To prevent bone loss, the adequate intake of vitamin D is doubled to 10 μg/d in men and women older than 50 years and tripled to 15 μg/d for adults older than 70 years compared with younger adults [28].

Calcium

Just as the need for vitamin D is increased for protection of bone health in older adults, so are calcium needs. The adequate intake has been established at 1200 mg/d for men and women older than 50 years. This recommendation is based on evidence that calcium absorption decreases with age. In addition, clinical trials in women older than 50 years have found that intakes greater than 1000 mg/d reduce bone loss [28]. Although there have been studies of varying intensities of physical activity on calcium needs, there is inconclusive evidence at this time that calcium needs should be adjusted for level of physical activity [28].

Vitamin B_6

Vitamin B_6 is involved in many metabolic pathways that produce energy during exercise. In the muscle, vitamin B_6 is necessary for the breakdown of glycogen in muscle, and it assists in converting lactic acid to glucose in the liver [29]. Research suggests that the requirements for vitamin B_6 are greater in adults older than 50 years. In addition, there is a gender difference in the vitamin requirement that does not exist in younger adults. Men older than 50 years should consume 1.7 mg/d, and women older than 50 years should consume 1.5 mg/d. Research on the need for vitamin B_6 in exercise is equivocal, and results are inconclusive to warrant changing the dietary requirement in exercising individuals [29].

Folate

Although aging does not seem to have an effect on folate absorption or use, it is a crucial nutrient for older adults. Research has found that low folate status is a risk factor for cognitive decline [31]. The mechanism by which this decline occurs seems to be through the methylation pathway of homocysteine metabolism. As a result of folate deficiency, the pathway is disturbed, and *S*-adenosylhomocysteine accumulates. The accumulation of *S*-adenosylhomocysteine inhibits methylation reactions, possibly resulting in cognitive dysfunction [31]. The RDA for folate for all adults is 400 μg/d of Dietary Folate Equivalents [30].

Vitamin B_{12}

It has been proposed that there is a decline in vitamin B_{12} status in older adults as plasma vitamin B_{12} levels decrease with age, and serum methylmalonic acid increases with age. There are several possible explanations for this decline with increasing age, including decreased gastric acidity, atrophic gastritis, bacterial overgrowth, malabsorption of food-bound vitamin B_{12}, lack of liver stores of vitamin B_{12}, and impaired binding proteins. Despite this evidence, the RDA for vitamin B_{12} for older adults is the same as for younger adults at 2.4 μg/d. For adults older than age 50, however, it is recommended that most vitamin B_{12} be obtained by consuming foods fortified with synthetic vitamin B_{12} or by taking a supplement containing vitamin B_{12} because the food-bound form is more difficult to absorb with aging [30].

Iron

Iron is the one micronutrient that is needed in lesser amounts for women after menopause. The RDA is reduced to 8 mg/d for women older than 50 years, which is the same level for men. For men and women who engage in regular, endurance exercise there is a greater loss of iron. In addition, decreased iron stores have been documented in athletes because iron has a shorter half-life in these individuals. A conservative estimate is that athletes need 30% more iron than individuals who do not exercise. No distinction has been made, however, with respect to the age of the athlete. It is possible that masters athletes may require 10.4 mg of iron a day [32].

Other Vitamins and Minerals

Regular and strenuous exercise may have an effect on thiamine, riboflavin, and choline, although more research is needed before specific recommendations can be made. There is limited evidence that thiamine requirements may be increased for individuals consistently engaged in active sports. Normal physical activity does not have a substantial effect, however, on thiamine needs. In addition, older adults may need more thiamine, although this may be compensated for by decreased energy expenditure. The current RDA of 1.2 mg/d for men and 1.1 mg/d for women is sufficient for masters athletes [30]. Similarly, riboflavin requirements may be increased for individuals who are very physically active, but there are no data to suggest how much is needed. The needs of older adults are no different from those of younger adults, so the RDA of 1.3 mg/d for men and 1.1 mg/d for women is adequate [30]. Plasma choline concentrations may be depleted as a result of strenuous exercise, although more research is needed to confirm this effect. There also may be reduced transport of choline across the blood-brain barrier in elderly individuals, which would suggest greater needs. At this time, however, the DRI is the same for older adults as younger at 550 mg/d for men and 425 mg/d for women [30].

Zinc has not been studied in relation to physical activity; however, it has been studied in elderly patients. It is possible that zinc metabolism is altered in older adults, but more research is needed before conclusions can be drawn. Aging does not have any negative effects on zinc absorption. The RDA for masters athletes is the same as for all adults at 11 mg/d for men and 8 mg/d for women [32]. Low zinc status has been linked to lower plasma total protein thiol groups in the exercising elderly. Oxidative stress immediately lowers plasma total protein thiol groups, and this could be even more pronounced in the exercising elderly if the DRI for zinc is not met [33].

Although studies have looked at the effect of exercise on magnesium levels, there is no clear evidence to suggest that exercise depletes magnesium stores in the body. In addition, research does not indicate a need for greater magnesium requirements in adults older than age 50. The recommended RDA of 420 mg/d for men and 320 mg/d for women is sufficient for masters athletes [28].

Antioxidants

Research has shown that exercise leads to oxidative stress in skeletal muscle through the production of lipid peroxides and free radicals. It has been postulated that antioxidants, which protect the body from cellular damage, may aid in recovery by reducing the damage of oxidative stress in skeletal muscle. Research shows that antioxidants may assist in recovery, although they do not have an effect on performance [34]. It also has been proposed that exercise enhances the body's response to oxidative stress by increasing the production of antioxidant enzymes [6]. It is unknown if the same response occurs in the exercising elderly as in young adults because few studies have focused on masters athletes. It is known, however, that regardless of exercise, oxidative stress increases with age. Rousseau and associates [33] conducted a study of the exercising elderly compared with sedentary counterparts and exercising and sedentary young adults. It was found that even high intakes of antioxidants coupled with exercise did not counteract the oxidative stress induced by advancing age, whereas antioxidant intake and exercise training were protective against oxidative damage in young athletes. Rousseau and associates [33] concluded that masters athletes have specific antioxidant requirements as they age, particularly for the carotenoids. Further research is warranted to explore these issues in depth.

Vitamin C

Several studies have looked at the vitamin C status of athletes. There is no evidence at this time that athletes require additional vitamin C greater than the RDA. In addition, advancing age has no effect on the absorption or metabolism of vitamin C. The RDA for men and women older than age 50 is 90 mg/d and 75 mg/d. Vitamin C supplementation is popular, and the Tolerable Upper Intake Level (UL) established in the DRIs at 2000 mg/d should be used as a guide for masters athletes [35].

Vitamin E

Vitamin E is another antioxidant that has been widely studied. Vitamin E may be beneficial in protecting the body from the oxidative stress resulting from exercise. There is not enough research at this time, however, to warrant a change in the requirements for athletes [33]. There is limited evidence that regular exercise in adults older than 60 years alters vitamin E status, but it is unknown whether requirements should be adjusted as a result of regular or strenuous exercise. There are currently no data to suggest that aging impairs the absorption or use of vitamin E. The RDA of 15 mg/d for adults older than age 50 is sufficient, regardless of activity level. The UL is set at 1000 mg/d and should be followed by masters athletes choosing to take supplements [35].

Carotenoids

There is not enough evidence at present to establish a DRI for beta-carotene and the other carotenoids; however, this does not diminish their importance in the diet. The current recommendation for older adults is to consume more carotenoid-rich fruits and vegetables. Beta-carotene supplements other than as a source of provitamin A to prevent vitamin A deficiency are not advised, however, because their potential to cause harm is great [35]. Research has found that plasma concentrations of lycopene, beta-carotene, and alpha-carotene were low in exercising elderly participants despite a high intake of these carotenoids [33]. Further research should be conducted to elucidate the carotenoid requirements of masters athletes.

Whole foods are the preferred source for the daily consumption of micronutrients. Although there is little research to suggest altering the DRI requirements for masters athletes, masters athletes should be striving to meet the DRI for all micronutrients through their diet. Research has shown that this is not the case, however. Nieman and coworkers [36] showed that female marathon runners are deficient in vitamin D and zinc. Chatard and colleagues [27] found that healthy Frenchmen between the ages of 57 and 72 who engaged in regular cycling, running, swimming, tennis, and walking did not meet the RDA for magnesium or vitamin D.

The use of supplements is popular, particularly among athletes. Supplement use can be the difference between masters athletes who meet the RDA and those that do not. In a study comparing the dietary intake of 25 female master cyclists and runners who took supplements versus those who did not, it was found that athletes who took supplements consumed significantly more vitamin C, vitamin E, calcium, and magnesium. On further analysis of dietary intake without accounting for the supplements, these same individuals consumed average levels below the RDA for vitamin D, vitamin E, folate, calcium, magnesium, and zinc [37]. For athletes taking supplements, the UL should be adhered to for all vitamins and minerals.

FLUID NEEDS

Hydration is crucial for all athletes, but masters athletes have to pay special attention to fluid intake. Aging brings physiologic changes to thirst sensation, sweating rates, renal adaptation to altered fluid and electrolyte status, and blood flow responses that can impair thermoregulation in older athletes [38]. Although no data are published to recommend a specific fluid plan or preferred beverages, guidelines for younger athletes can be used to establish a fluid plan for masters athletes. Assessing the athlete's daily fluid intake and monitoring intake during training and competition can establish a baseline for developing a hydration strategy [39].

SUMMARY

Very little is known about the nutrient intakes, nutritional status, or nutritional needs of masters athletes. As the population ages and more people remain physically active and engaged in competitive sports in later life, more research is needed to identify nutritional strategies to fuel these athletes.

References

[1] US athletes to compete at 2006 World Masters Athletes Championships Indoor. News release 3–15–06. Available at: http://www.usatf.org/news. Accessed April 15, 2006.
[2] Huntsman World Senior Games. Available at: http://www.hwsg.com/Archives/media.html. Accessed April 15, 2006.
[3] National Senior Games. Available at: http://www.nsga.org. Accessed April 20, 2006.
[4] Harrison D. Have aging athletes found the fountain of youth? CBC Sports Online. Available at: http://www.cbc.ca/sports/columns/analysis/harrison/harrison_050301.html. Accessed March 30, 2006.
[5] Press Room. Did you know? Department of Health and Human Services, Administration on Aging. Available at: http://www.aoa.gov/press/did_you_know/did_you_know.asp?pf=true. Accessed March 30, 2006.
[6] 38 Million boomers to be 50+: insights to help you tap this trillion dollar market. New York: FIND/SVP, Inc; 2002.
[7] Seals DR, Allen WK, Hurley BF, et al. Elevated high-density lipoprotein cholesterol levels in older endurance athletes. Am J Cardiol 1984;54:390–3.
[8] Seals DR, Hagberg JM, Allen WK, et al. Glucose tolerance in young and older athletes and sedentary men. J Appl Physiol 1984;56:1521–5.
[9] Etherington J, Harris PA, Nandra D, et al. The effect of weight-bearing exercise on bone mineral density: a study of female ex-athletes and the general population. J Bone Miner Res 1996;11:1333–8.
[10] Morgan WP, Costill DL. Selected psychological characteristics and health behaviors of aging marathon runners: a longitudinal study. Int J Sports Med 1996;17:305–12.
[11] Rosenbloom CA. Masters athletes. In: Dunford M, editor. Sports nutrition: a practice manual for professionals. 4th edition. Chicago: American Dietetic Association; 2006. p. 269–82.
[12] Rosenbloom CA, Bahns M. What can we learn about diet and physical activity from master athletes? Nutr Today 2005;40:267–72.
[13] Starling RD. Energy expenditure and aging: effects of physical activity. Int J Sports Nutr Exerc Metab 2001;11:S208–17.
[14] Wilson MMG, Morley JE. Invited review: aging and energy balance. J Appl Physiol 2003;95:1729–36.
[15] Van Pelt RE, Jones PP, Davy KP, et al. Regular exercise and the age-related decline in resting metabolic rate in women. J Clin Endocrinol Metab 1997;82:3208–12.
[16] van Pelt RE, Dinneno FA, Seals DR, et al. Age-related decline in RMR in physically active men: relation to exercise volume and energy intake. Am J Physiol Endrocrinol Metab 2001;281(3):E633–9.
[17] Simkin-Silverman LR, Wing RR. Weight gain during menopause. Postgrad Med 2000;108: 4–56.
[18] Holcomb CA, Heim DL, Loughin TM. Physical activity minimizes the association of body fatness with abdominal obesity in white, premenopausal women: results from the Third National Health and Nutrition Examination Survey. J Am Diet Assoc 2004;104: 1859–62.

[19] Institute of Medicine. Dietary Reference Intakes for energy, carbohydrates, fiber, fat, protein and amino acids (macronutrients). Washington, DC: National Academy Press; 2002. Available at: http://www.nap.edu/books. Accessed March 30, 2006.
[20] Coleman EJ. Carbohydrate and exercise. In: Dunford M, editor. Sports nutrition: a practice manual for professionals. 4th edition. Chicago: American Dietetic Association; 2006. p. 14–32.
[21] Roubenoff R, Castaneda C. Sarcopenia—understanding the dynamics of aging muscle. JAMA 2001;286:1230–1.
[22] Doherty TJ. Invited review: aging and sarcopenia. J Appl Physiol 2003;95:1717–27.
[23] Meredith CN, Zacklin WR, Frontera WR, et al. Dietary protein requirements and body protein metabolism in endurance-trained men. J Appl Physiol 1989;66:2850–6.
[24] Campbell WW, Crim MC, Young VR, et al. Effects of resistance training and dietary protein intake on protein metabolism in older adults. Am J Physiol 1995;268:E1143–53.
[25] Gibala MJ, Howarth KR. Protein and exercise. In: Dunford M, editor. Sports nutrition: a practice manual for professionals. 4th edition. Chicago: American Dietetic Association; 2006. p. 33–49.
[26] American Dietetic Association. Position of the American Dietetic Association, Dietitians of Canada, and the American College of Sports Medicine: nutrition and athletic performance. J Am Diet Assoc 2000;100:1543–56.
[27] Chatard JC, Boutet C, Tourny C, et al. Nutritional status and physical fitness of elderly sportsmen. Eur J Appl Physiol 1998;77:157–63.
[28] Institute of Medicine, Food and Nutrition Board. Dietary Reference Intakes for calcium, phosphorus, magnesium, vitamin D and fluoride. Washington, DC: National Academy Press; 1997.
[29] Manore MM. Effect of physical activity on thiamine, riboflavin, and vitamin B-6 requirements. Am J Clin Nutr 2000;72(Suppl):598S–606S.
[30] Institute of Medicine, Food and Nutrition Board. Dietary Reference Intakes for thiamin, riboflavin, niacin, vitamin B6, folate, vitamin B12, pantothenic acid, biotin, and choline. Washington, DC: National Academy Press; 1998.
[31] Kado DM, Karlamangla AS, Huang MH, et al. Homocysteine versus the vitamins folate, B6, and B12 as predictors of cognitive function and decline in older high-functioning adults: MacArthur Studies of Successful Aging. Am J Med 2005;118:161–7.
[32] Institute of Medicine, Food and Nutrition Board. Dietary Reference Intakes for vitamin A, vitamin K, arsenic, boron, chromium, copper, iodine, iron, manganese, molybdenum, nickel, silicon, vanadium and zinc. Washington, DC: National Academy Press; 2001.
[33] Rousseau AS, Margaritis I, Arnaud J, et al. Physical activity alters antioxidant status in exercising elderly subjects. J Nutr Biochem 2006;17(7):463–70.
[34] Berning JR. Nutrition for exercise and sports performance. In: Mahan LK, Escott-Stump S, editors. Krause's food, nutrition and diet therapy. 11th edition. Philadelphia: Saunders; 2004. p. 616–41.
[35] Institute of Medicine, Food and Nutrition Board. Dietary Reference Intakes for vitamin C, vitamin E, selenium, and carotenoids. Washington, DC: National Academy Press; 2000.
[36] Nieman DC, Butler JC, Pollett LM, et al. Nutrient intake of marathon runners. J Am Diet Assoc 1989;89:1273–8.
[37] Beshgetoor D, Nichols JF. Dietary intake and supplement use in female master cyclists and runners. Int J Sport Nutr Exerc Metab 2003;13:166–72.
[38] Kenney WL. Are there special hydration requirements for older individuals engaged in exercise? Aust J Nutr Dietetics 1996;53:S43–4.
[39] Crosland J. Nutrition across the year. The Coach 2004;23:49–51.

Clin Sports Med 26 (2007) 101–118

CLINICS IN SPORTS MEDICINE

ELSEVIER
SAUNDERS

Nutritional Considerations in Joint Health

Kristine L. Clark, PhD, RD

Pennsylvania State University, Room 256, Recreation Hall, University Park, PA 16802, USA

Osteoarthritis, a debilitating joint disorder, is the most common form of arthritis in the United States [1], where it affects an estimated 21 million people. In 2004, the direct and indirect health care costs associated with all forms of arthritis were approximately $86 billion [2]. Joint discomfort from osteoarthritis and other joint disorders may reduce physical activity in individuals experiencing this condition, resulting in energy imbalance and weight gain. Increased weight can exacerbate existing problems, as additional stress on joints stimulates risk of additional joint disorders. Dietitians play a role in preventing or reversing the problem of joint disorders by promoting nutrient-rich diets that support joint health through improvement in cartilage metabolism. In addition, counseling individuals on weight management and active lifestyles are key strategies for the management of joint health.

JOINT

Joints are structures in the body that provide movement and mechanical support [3]. Although there are several types of joints in the human body, this article focuses on synovial joints, such as those in the knees, arms, and shoulders. These joints, found at the ends of bones, have a space that allows for a wide range of motion [3]. Formed by endochondral ossification, joints are strengthened by a dense fibrous capsule that is reinforced by ligaments and muscles [3]. The capsule is filled with synovial fluid, a clear liquid that contains hyaluronic acid, a lubricant that also provides nutrients to the joint tissues [3].

The surfaces where two bones meet are covered with articular cartilage. Articular cartilage consists of four layers of tissue (Fig. 1). First, a thin superficial layer provides a smooth surface for two bones to slide against each other. The second layer is very resistant to shear stresses. An intermediate layer is mechanically designed to absorb shock and distribute load or weight efficiently. The fourth or deepest layer is highly calcified and anchors the articular cartilage to the bone.

A unique aspect of articular cartilage is the isolation of its component cells from each other and from other cell types. It is one of the few tissues in the

E-mail address: klc5@psu.edu

0278-5919/07/$ – see front matter
doi:10.1016/j.csm.2006.11.006

© 2007 Elsevier Inc. All rights reserved.

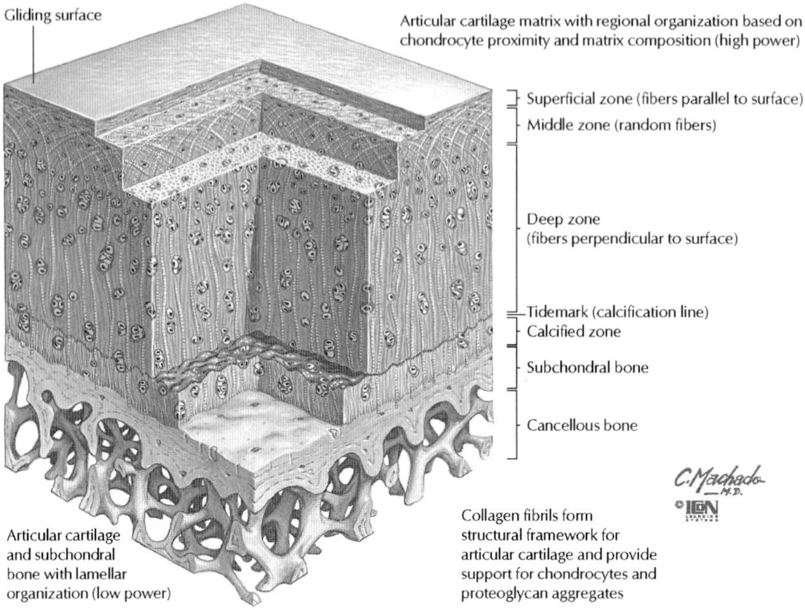

Fig. 1. Layers of cartilage in a joint. (Courtesy of Netter Images. Available at: www.NetterImages.com.)

human body that does not have its own blood supply. It obtains its nutrition principally from diffusion of synovial fluid in the synovial cavity [4].

Articular cartilage is able to provide support and flexibility because of the structure of its extracellular matrix [5]. This matrix contains proteoglycans, which are responsible for the compressive stiffness of the tissue and its ability to withstand load, and type 2 collagen, which provides tensile strength and resistance to shear [6], water, chondrocytes, and other molecules [3]. The collagen fibers are arranged in arches, a horizontal orientation near the surface of the cartilage. This orientation allows the cartilage to resist stress and to transmit weight [3].

The water and proteoglycans provide cartilage with elasticity and play a crucial role in reducing friction. Most proteoglycans in articular cartilage are in the form of aggrecan, aggregates of proteoglycan monomers bound to a hyaluronic acid backbone by a noncovalent association with a link glycoprotein. The highly charged, polysulfated glycosaminoglycan components of the aggrecan molecules attract cations and water, resulting in osmotic pressure in the tissue owing to the constraint of the molecular configuration caused by containment within the collagen meshwork [7].

The chondrocytes maintain a balance between production and degradation of cartilage extracellular matrix [3]. Matrix turnover is modulated by chondrocytes that secrete degradative enzymes and enzyme inhibitors [3]. The number and activity of chondrocytes affect the anatomic and tribologic features of cartilage [8]. The chondrocyte itself is regulated by various cytokines and growth factors that can alter the homeostatic balance toward an anabolic or catabolic direction [9,10].

Most load on articular cartilage is produced by contraction of the muscles that stabilize and move the joints [6]. Although cartilage is an excellent shock absorber, it is usually 1 to 2 mm thick in most parts of the joint, which is too thin to serve as the only shock-absorbing tissue in the joint. Subchondral bone and periarticular muscles provide additional protective effects [6].

BASIC NUTRITIONAL REQUIREMENTS OF HEALTHY JOINTS

A balanced, nutritionally adequate diet is required to maintain healthy joints (Box 1). Key nutrients include the following:

- *Calcium.* The adult body contains about 1200 g of calcium, approximately 99% of which is present in the skeleton. Bone mineral consists of two chemically and physically distinct calcium phosphate pools—an amorphous phase and a loosely crystallized phase. The skeleton contains two major forms of bone: trabecular (spongy) bone and cortical (dense) bone, both of which constantly turn over in a continuous process of resorption (loss) and reformation (gain). In later life, resorption predominates over formation. Growth of bone requires a positive calcium balance. Peak bone mass seems to be related to intake of calcium during the years of bone mineralization. The age at which peak bone mass is attained is uncertain, but probably is not less than 25 years. The recommendation for optimal bone formation is consumption of 1200 mg/d of calcium for males and females between the ages of 11 and 24 years. For optimal maintenance of bone mineral density with aging, 1500 mg has been suggested. Dairy products or foods fortified with calcium offer the best sources of calcium along with additional nutrients, such as lactose, vitamin D, and phosphorus, which seem to support calcium absorption.
- *Phosphorus.* This nutrient is an essential component of bone mineral. Approximately 85% of all phosphorus in the body is found in the skeleton. Major contributors of phosphorus in the food supply are protein-rich foods such as milk, meat, fish, and poultry. Cereal grains provide about 12% of dietary phosphorus, whereas diets based heavily on processed foods receive an additional 20% to 30% of phosphorus from food additives. Recommended intakes for

Box 1: Nutrients required for healthy joints

- Calcium (from dairy products, fish bones)
- Vitamin D (from milk, sunlight)
- Phosphorus (from citrus fruits, juices, vegetables)
- Protein (from milk, eggs, meats, fish, grains, vegetables, beans, nuts, seeds)
- Zinc (from lean red meat, pork, the dark meat of chicken, whole-grain cereals, and dairy products such as milk and cheese)

phosphorus are 800 mg/d for children between the ages of 1 and 10 years, 1200 mg/d for individuals 11 to 24 years, and 800 mg/d for individuals older than 24 years old. Dietary phosphorus is more abundant than calcium in most US diets.

- *Protein.* Overall, protein's role in healthy joint formation is its contribution of amino acids and nitrogen for growth. Without adequate protein, optimal bone and joint formation is compromised. Especially important are sulfur-containing amino acids, such as the nonessential amino acid cysteine, which contributes sulfur. In animal studies, there have been reports of reduced levels of sulfur in joints associated with osteoarthritis [11].
- *Vitamin C.* Ascorbic acid stimulates collagen synthesis and modestly stimulates synthesis of aggrecan [12].
- *Vitamin D.* Normal bone and cartilage metabolism depends on the presence of vitamin D [13]. Suboptimal levels of vitamin D are reported to cause adverse effects on articular cartilage turnover. In tissue culture, vitamin D has been shown to have a direct effect on the synthesis of proteoglycan by chondrocytes [14]. In addition, researchers have shown that dietary intake of vitamin D in patients with osteoarthritis is less than 80% of the recommended daily allowance [15]. In the Framingham study comprising 556 participants, the risk of osteoarthritis progression increased threefold in participants in the middle and lower tertiles for vitamin D intake and serum levels of vitamin D [16].
- *Vitamin E.* Research suggests that vitamin E may enhance chondrocyte growth, provide protection against reactive oxygen species, and modulate the development of osteoarthritis [17,18]. It has been shown that many osteoarthritis patients have dietary intakes of vitamin E that are below the recommended daily allowance of 400 IU/d [19].
- *Zinc.* Low zinc levels have been reported in patients with osteoarthritis [15,19,20]. The recommended daily allowance for zinc in males is 11 mg, whereas for females it is 8 mg. Vegetarians may need 50% more zinc than nonvegetarians, owing to decreased absorption of zinc from plant sources.

In addition to these nutrients, healthy joints require that individuals get adequate levels of collagenous materials in their diet. Collagen naturally occurs in the gristle of meats. Recommendations to reduce meat consumption, which aim to reduce saturated fat and decrease risk for cardiovascular disease, have increased speculation that the amount of collagen in the average Western diet may be declining. Many consumers prefer lean, boneless meats without connective tissue. The adoption of lactovegetarianism also may reduce the amount of collagen in the diet. Concerns about bovine spongiform encephalopathy, commonly known as mad cow disease, also have contributed to a decline in the consumption of meat, which may have resulted in decreased collagen consumption. While essential nutrients for joint health may be decreasing, there is a concomitant increase in obesity and overweight, putting additional stress or overload on joints.

JOINT DISORDERS

Causes of Joint Problems

Athletic activities can influence joint problems from a variety of different causes. Joint problems can arise from normal use in individuals with existing joint diseases or from overuse or excessive stress specific to a sport (eg, joint pain from running or cycling or constant repetitive stress on a specific knee). These causes including the following:

- *Stress (microfractures, osteochondrophytes).* Many activities, including sports-related activities, cause excess stress on joints, which leads to microfractures in the surrounding bone. This damage can lead to the formation of osteochondrophytes and calluses that cause thickening of the joint area.
- *Dietary habits.* Two aspects of dietary habits can affect joint health: an early-in-life deficiency of nutrients necessary for optimal bone and joint formation and overconsumption of total calories (resulting in overweight or obesity). In Western societies, excess caloric intake is more likely to be a problem than early deficiency of nutrients.
- *Injury and trauma.* Power and contact sports with a high risk of injury increase the risk of severe degenerative disease of the joints involved.
- *Disease.* The most common type of joint disease is osteoarthritis [3,6]. Although the term *osteoarthritis* suggests an inflammatory disease, osteoarthritis is a disease of the synovial joint, in which all of the tissues are affected, including the subchondral bone, synovium, meniscus, ligaments, supporting neuromuscular apparatus, and cartilage, in which biochemical and metabolic alterations result in the breakdown of this tissue. Some inflammatory cells may be present in osteoarthritis, but inflammation is not the primary disease state [3]. It is believed that degeneration of cartilage in osteoarthritis is characterized by two phases: a biosynthetic phase, during which the chondrocytes in cartilage attempt to repair damage to the extracellular matrix, and a degradative phase, in which the activity of enzymes produced by the chondrocytes digest the matrix, matrix synthesis is inhibited, and the consequent erosion of cartilage is accelerated [21–24].
- *Obesity.* Although there are conflicting data on the linear, causal correlation between overweight and the frequency and severity of joint disease, it is generally accepted that degenerative joint disease occurs more frequently in obese individuals [25–27]. Coggon and associates [27] reported that the risk of osteoarthritis of the knee increased from 0.1 with a body mass index (BMI) of less than 20 kg/m^2 to 13.6 for a BMI of 36 kg/m^2 or greater. In addition, it has been reported that if overweight and obese individuals reduced their weight by 5 kg or until their BMI was within the recommended normal range, 24% of surgical cases of knee osteoarthritis would be avoided [27]. Some researchers have suggested that the increased risk of joint problems is not only the added mechanical stress brought about by overweight, but also the metabolic disturbance associated with obesity that has an additional effect on cartilage metabolism. This view is supported by evidence that osteoarthritis of the fingers, which is not associated with mechanical stress, seems to occur more frequently in obese individuals [28–30].
- *Aging.* By age 70, most adults have some form of osteoarthritic joint disease. Although not specifically a result of aging, it may be due to the fact that many elderly individuals have a generalized vitamin deficiency [31].
- *Congenital deformity.* Another cause of joint disorders is skeletal deformity and joint malposition. In such cases, uneven stress from the deformed or misaligned joint causes the cartilage tissue to be worn down or injured over time.

PREVENTING AND ADDRESSING JOINT DISORDERS

Currently, there is no cure for joint disorders such as osteoarthritis, so treatment focuses on reducing pain and inflammation with the goal of maintaining mobility and avoiding unnecessary stress to the painful joint area. Management strategies include exercise, reduction in weight, and nonpharmacologic and pharmacologic interventions.

Lifestyle Treatments: Exercise, Stretching, Aerobic Activity, and Weight Management

Targeted and well-dosed physical stress helps keep avascular cartilage supplied with nutrients and free to metabolize waste products. Because of this and other factors, a physically active lifestyle is an important aspect of the complex treatment of joint disorders [32]. Various kinds of therapy are recommended for treating joint disorders, including functional training; isometric, isotonic, and isokinetic exercises; postural training; and general strengthening exercises [33–37]. Stretching exercises are important to help muscles, tendons, and ligaments retain strength and ensure that no further restrictions in mobility develop [32]. Exercises should be moderate in nature to prevent stress to the joints. In addition, relaxation is important (at least 4–6 hours each day).

Dietary Treatments: Optimal Nutrition

Maintaining healthy joints starts with adequate nutrition. Athletes should get adequate levels of protein to maintain and repair muscles, tendons, ligaments, and joints. Fruits and vegetables provide antioxidants that can help reduce inflammation and improve recovery from and adaptation to exercise. Essential fats, especially omega-3 fatty acids, are beneficial for promoting prostaglandins that control inflammation and pain pathways. Some essential fatty acids, such as omega-6 fatty acids, are easy to obtain from dietary sources because they are readily available in plant oils. A 1:1 or 2:1 ratio of omega-6 to omega-3 fats in the daily diet has been suggested. The amount of omega-3 fatty acids can be achieved by eating fish two to three times per week and using flax oil regularly.

In animal studies, high levels of vitamin C (150 mg/d) in the diet resulted in less severe joint damage in guinea pigs with surgically induced osteoarthritis compared with guinea pigs receiving low levels (2.4 mg/d) [38,39]. In the Framingham Osteoarthritis Cohort Study, a moderate intake of vitamin C (120–200 mg/d) resulted in a threefold lower risk of osteoarthritis progression, but did not have an impact on the incidence of the disease [40]. A multicenter, double-blind, randomized, placebo-controlled, crossover trial was conducted on 133 patients with radiographically verified symptomatic osteoarthritis of the hip or knee joints. The patients received 1 g of calcium ascorbate (containing 898 mg of vitamin C) or placebo daily for 14 ± 3 days, separated by 7 ± 3 days washout. Calcium ascorbate was reported to reduce pain significantly compared with placebo, although the demonstrated effect was less than half that commonly reported with nonsteroidal anti-inflammatory drugs (NSAIDs) [41].

Clinical studies have reported benefits from vitamin E administered for the treatment of symptomatic osteoarthritis over a short-term period [42–44]. Two large studies, performed over a longer period, found no evidence of benefits in terms of reduced pain or stiffness or improved physical function [45,46].

Nonpharmacologic and Pharmacologic Treatments

No medications have been shown to reverse the damage to joints caused by injury or disease, so pain relief is the main goal for individuals with osteoarthritis and other joint disorders. Many patients with joint pain use NSAIDs [47]. On average, 30% pain relief and 15% functional improvement have been reported [6]. Although NSAIDs may suppress inflammation, they do not improve the natural history of the disease. Another problem with NSAIDs is that they are associated with an increased risk of side effects, including the following [48]:

- Epigastric discomfort
- Gastric or duodenal ulcers
- Gastrointestinal bleeding
- Exacerbation of the degenerative process of osteoarthritis by decreasing production of glycosaminoglycan synthesis

Another class of medications for the treatment of joint pain is the cyclooxygenase-2 (COX-2) inhibitors, which target COX-2, an enzyme responsible for inflammation and pain [49]. COX-2 inhibitors were associated with fewer gastrointestinal side effects than the NSAIDs in several large studies [50,51]. Concerns about cardiovascular effects led to the COX-2 inhibitor rofecoxib being withdrawn from the market on September 30, 2004, however [52].

The systemic administration of glucocorticoids is another approach to joint pain used by some clinicians. This approach is not considered effective for osteoarthritis. Depot glucocorticoids may have a pain-reducing effect over many weeks if given by intra-articular or periarticular injection [53,54]. Although this approach is recommended in several guidelines for the management of patients with peripheral joint osteoarthritis [55,56], the long-term effect of treatment on cartilage metabolism and the progression of osteoarthritis is unclear [57]. A specialist should administer intra-articular injections, and they should be given at most two or three times per year to the same joint.

SUPPLEMENTS AND HERBS FOR OPTIMIZING JOINT HEALTH

Herbal Products

Various herbal products have been studied for the treatment of joint disorders, including green tea extracts, Asian herbal remedies (eg, *Tripterygium wilfordi* Hook F, SKI 306X [a mixture of extracts from *Clematis mandshurica, Tricosanthes kirilowii,* and *Prunella vulgaris*]), and devil's claw (*Harpagophytum procumbens*) [58].

- Green tea contains polyphenolic compounds called catechins [58]. The catechins in green tea include (−)-epigallocatechin 3-gallate (EGCG), (−)-epigallocatechin, (−)-epicatechin 3-gallate (ECG), and (−)-epicatechin [58]. A polyphenolic fraction from green tea has been reported to prevent collagen-induced arthritis in mice [59]. In a study that used a bovine in vitro model of cartilage degradation, EGCG and ECG were shown to inhibit interleukin (IL)-1–induced proteoglycan release and type II collagen degradation in cartilage explants [60]. In a human in vitro model, EGCG was shown to suppress IL-1β-induced inducible nitric oxide synthase mRNA and protein expression and the production of nitric oxide [61]. Further studies are required, however, to determine whether oral consumption of green tea can result in sufficiently high concentrations of catechins in joints to provide the same effects seen in the in vitro studies [58].

- Tao and colleagues [62] reported the effects of a Chinese herbal medicine called *Tripterygium wilfordii* Hook F in a clinical trial using patients with rheumatoid arthritis. They found that an extract of the plant suppressed symptoms of rheumatoid arthritis compared with a placebo control.
- The compound SKI 306X (an herbal product extracted from the herbs *Clematis mandshurica, Trichosanthes kirilowii,* and *Prunella vulgaris*) has been reported to inhibit IL-1-induced proteoglycan degradation in rabbit articular cartilage explants and to decrease lesions in a collagen-induced osteoarthritis model in rabbits [63]. The complex nature of these extracts and their variability has prevented elucidation of the active ingredients in this compound, however, and their specific mechanisms of action [58].
- Extracts of the root of devil's claw (*Harpagophytum procumbens*), a plant originally found in the savannas of South West Africa, is believed to have anti-inflammatory and analgesic effects, which may be associated with its component harpagoside [64]. A review of the literature concluded that there is some evidence that *Harpagophytum* powder containing 60 mg of harpagoside provides some relief to patients with osteoarthritis of the spine, knee, and hip [65].

Glucosamine Sulfate and Chondroitin Sulfate

Glucosamine sulfate and chondroitin sulfate supplements are the most widely used dietary supplements for the treatment of osteoarthritis, with an annual sales of nearly $730 million in 2004 [66]. Glucosamine is an amino monosaccharide that is the most fundamental building block required for the biosynthesis of several classes of compounds that require amino sugars, such as glycosaminoglycans and proteoglycans [67]. The raw material for glucosamine is derived from chitin, a biopolymer present in the exoskeleton of marine invertebrate animals [68]. Chondroitin sulfates are a class of glycosaminoglycans required for the formation of proteoglycans found in joint cartilage [67].

The rationale for the use of glucosamine and chondroitin is based on the assertion that osteoarthritis is associated with a local deficiency in some key nutritional substances, and that providing these substances addresses this deficiency and supports cartilage repair [58,69]. Glucosamine sulfate has been shown to be capable of stimulating proteoglycan synthesis and regeneration of cartilage in animals after experimentally induced damage and inhibiting the degradation of proteoglycans [70,71]. It also has been suggested that chondroitin sulfate may increase proteoglycan synthesis and inhibit the activity of degradative enzymes [72,73].

Clinical research with glucosamine sulfate and chondroitin sulfate

Numerous clinical trials have tested the efficacy of glucosamine sulfate and chondroitin sulfate to reduce pain and provide functional improvement in patients with joint disorders, such as osteoarthritis. These studies were evaluated in a meta-analysis by McAlindon and colleagues [74], who reviewed 15 placebo-controlled glucosamine or chondroitin trials. The authors of the meta-analysis reported that trials of glucosamine and chondroitin preparations for the management of osteoarthritis symptoms showed moderate-to-large effects, but that quality issues and likely publication bias suggest that these effects are exaggerated [74].

GAIT trial

Many of the design flaws of glucosamine sulfate and chondroitin sulfate studies, including the failure to adhere to the intention-to-treat principle, the enrollment of small numbers of patients, potential bias because of sponsorship by a manufacturer of dietary supplements, and inadequate masking of the study agent, were addressed in the GAIT (Glucosamine/chondroitin Arthritis Intervention Trial), a study sponsored by the National Institutes of Health [1]. In GAIT, Clegg and coworkers [1] investigated glucosamine sulfate, chondroitin sulfate, and the two supplements in combination in a multicenter, double-blind, placebo-controlled and celecoxib-controlled study with 1583 patients with symptomatic knee osteoarthritis who were randomly assigned to receive 1500 mg of glucosamine sulfate daily, 1200 mg of chondroitin sulfate daily, both glucosamine sulfate and chondroitin sulfate, 200 mg of celecoxib daily, or placebo for 24 weeks. Up to 4000 mg of acetaminophen daily was allowed as rescue analgesia. The mean age of the patients was 59 years, and 64% were women [1]. The primary outcome measure was a 20% decrease in knee pain from baseline to week 24.

The investigators reported that glucosamine sulfate and chondroitin sulfate were not statistically significantly better than placebo in reducing knee pain by 20% (the primary outcome they had defined) [1]. Compared with the rate of response to placebo, the rate of response to glucosamine sulfate was 3.9% higher ($P = .30$), the rate of response to chondroitin sulfate was 5.3% higher ($P = .17$), and the rate of response to combined treatment was 6.5% higher ($P = .09$), whereas the response in the celecoxib control group was 10% higher ($P = .008$) (Fig. 2) [1]. The investigators concluded that glucosamine sulfate and chondroitin sulfate alone or in combination did not reduce pain effectively in the overall group of patients with osteoarthritis of the knee [1].

Methylsulfonylmethane

Methylsulfonylmethane (MSM) is another dietary supplement that is taken for the treatment of joint pain from arthritis. Its benefits for patients with osteoarthritis were investigated in a randomized, double-blind, placebo-controlled trial with 50 men and women (40–76 years old) with pain from osteoarthritis of the knee who were enrolled in an outpatient medical center [75]. The patients received MSM 3 g or placebo twice each day (6 g/d) for 12 weeks. The outcomes included the Western Ontario and McMaster University Osteoarthritis Index visual analog scale (WOMAC), patient and physician global assessments, and SF-36 (an overall health-related quality-of-life measurement).

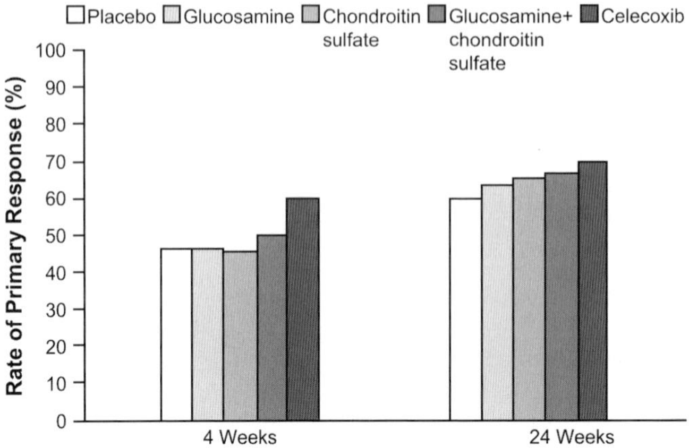

Fig. 2. Rates of primary response in the five groups in GAIT at 4 and 24 weeks. A primary response was defined as a 20% decrease in the summed score for the pain subscale of the WOMAC index. (*From* Clegg DO, Reda DJ, Harris CL, et al. Glucosamine, chondroitin sulfate, and the two in combination for painful knee osteoarthritis. N Engl J Med 2006;354:795–808; with permission.)

The investigators reported that MSM resulted in significantly decreased WOMAC pain and physical function impairment ($P < .05$) compared with placebo, but no notable changes were found in WOMAC stiffness and aggregated total symptom scores [75]. MSM also produced improvement in performing activities of daily living compared with placebo on the SF-36 evaluation ($P < .05$). They concluded that MSM (3 g twice a day) improved symptoms of pain and physical function during a short intervention without major adverse events, although the long-term benefits and safety in managing osteoarthritis could not be confirmed by this pilot trial [75].

S-Adenosyl-L-methionine

The dietary supplement *S*-adenosyl-L-methionine (SAMe) has been reported to be effective for the management of a variety of problems, including depression, liver disease, and arthritis [76]. It has been suggested that SAMe can reduce pain in osteoarthritis because it reduces inflammation, increases proteoglycan synthesis, or has an analgesic effect [76]. It is unknown whether SAMe is an inhibitor of COX-2. Studies using human articular chondrocytes have shown SAMe-induced increases in proteoglycan synthesis [77]. A double-blind crossover study compared SAMe (1200 mg) with celecoxib (Celebrex; 200 mg) for 16 weeks to reduce pain associated with osteoarthritis of the knee. Sixty-one adults diagnosed with osteoarthritis of the knee were enrolled, and 56 completed the study. The investigators reported that SAMe had a slower onset of action, but was as effective as celecoxib in the management of symptoms of knee osteoarthritis [76]. They concluded that longer studies are needed to determine the long-term efficacy of SAMe and the optimal dose to be used.

Collagen Hydrolysate

Collagen is a vital component of structural matrix throughout most tissues and organs in the human body. It is concentrated in cartilage, where it plays a significant role in the integrity of joint-related connective tissues. The important role played by collagen in joints is vividly shown by the severe generalized arthritis associated with collagen gene mutations [78,79].

The amount of collagen in the diet can be increased by consuming specific foods, such as meats with gristle or connective tissue still intact. Collagen also can be found in foods containing gelatin. Dietary supplements also can be used to increase the amount of collagen contributed by the diet. An example of such a supplement is collagen hydrolysate, which is prepared by enzymatic hydrolysis of collagenous tissue, such as bone, hide, and hide split from pigs and cows. Collagen hydrolysate is soluble in cold water and is composed of proteins with a molecular weight of 3 to 6 kD.

Collagen hydrolysate provides high levels of amino acids. Among these are glycine and proline, two amino acids that are essential for the stability and regeneration of cartilage. To synthesize a single picogram of collagen type II, more than 1 billion glycine molecules and 620 million proline molecules are required. In the absence of these amino acids, the anabolic phase of cartilage metabolism can be impaired.

In studies of rats and humans, concentrations of the amino acids proline, hydroxyproline, and glycine after administration of collagen hydrolysate (10 g in humans) increased significantly compared with placebo [80]. In a single-blind, randomized, and placebo-controlled study of 60 male sports students, the amino acid concentrations in peripheral blood after a daily intake of 10 g of collagen hydrolysate for 4.5 months were measured. It was found that levels of the amino acids glycine, proline, and hydroxyproline were significantly higher in the treated group than in the control group. The concentrations of alanine, asparagine, glutamic acid, and tryptophan also were higher.

Mechanism of action

It has been shown that about 90% of orally administered collagen hydrolysate is resorbed within 6 hours from the gastrointestinal tract [81]. It also has been found that collagen hydrolysate has a special affinity for cartilage, and that this affinity to cartilage has a stimulating effect on the synthesis of chondrocytes (Fig. 3) [81].

Clinical research on collagen hydrolysate

Collagen hydrolysate has been studied for the management of joint pain in four open-label and three double-blind studies [82–88]. The earliest of these, by Krug [82], studied the clinical effect of collagen hydrolysate on degenerative joint disease in patients with knee osteoarthritis with tibial, femoral, or retropatellar involvement or with degenerative disc disease of specific parts of the spine. Patients received 5 to 7 g of collagen hydrolysate by mouth for 1 to 6 months. The author reported results on 56 patients: 10 (24%) had very good success, 18 (44%) had noticeable improvement, and 13 (32%) reported no improvement. The author did not report the statistical significance of the findings [82].

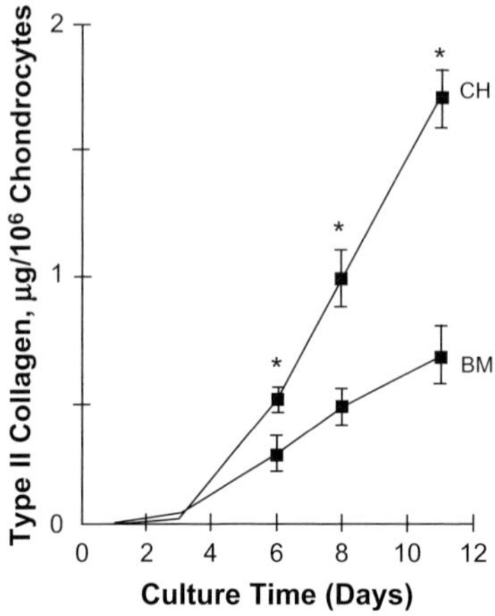

Fig. 3. Time course of type II collagen biosynthesis of chondrocytes cultured in basal medium (BM) or in medium supplemented with collagen hydrolysate (CH). *$P<.01$ compared with untreated controls. (*From* Oesser S, Seifert J. Stimulation of type II collagen biosynthesis and secretion in bovine chondrocytes cultured with degraded collagen. Cell Tissue Res 2003;311: 393–9; with kind permission of Springer Science and Business Media.)

In 1982, Götz [83] reported the results of a study in which 60 juvenile patients diagnosed with retropatellar osteoarthritis received collagen hydrolysate treatment (one 7-g sachet per day by mouth) for 3 months. The sachet also included 24,000 U of vitamin A and 120 mg of the sulfur-containing amino acid L-cysteine. Götz [83] reported that after treatment, 75% of patients showed improvement: 45% of patients were symptom-free, and 30% had clearly improved symptoms; the remainder of the patients did not improve. No *P* values were provided in this report.

An open-label study of 154 patients with osteoarthritis provided additional evidence of the clinical efficacy of collagen hydrolysate [84]. Patients with diagnosed osteoarthritis of the knee, hip, or lower spine were randomized among three treatment groups: therapeutic exercises; therapeutic exercises plus collagen hydrolysate with vitamin A and L-cysteine; or collagen hydrolysate, vitamin A, and L-cysteine without therapeutic exercise. The collagen hydrolysate, vitamin A, and L-cysteine were given as one sachet per day by mouth. After 3 months of treatment, the percentage of patients with a very good response was 26% for the supplement-only group, 20% for the supplement plus exercise group, and 6% for the exercise-only group [84]. Similar results were found for good response (supplement only, 43%; supplement plus exercise, 36%; and exercise only, 14%), whereas the opposite results were found for patients who were considered unchanged (supplement only, 6%; supplement plus exercise, 14%; and exercise only, 43%).

Collagen hydrolysate has been studied in populations other than patients diagnosed with osteoarthritis. An observational study investigated the effects of collagen hydrolysate in athletes who had joint pain, but who did not have osteoarthritis. In this study, 100 participants with hip, knee, or shoulder pain resulting from intense physical activity were treated with orally administered collagen hydrolysate (10 g/d) for 12 weeks [87]. Of the 88 patients who could be evaluated in the study, 78% of patients achieved pain reduction after taking collagen hydrolysate for 12 weeks (68 patients improved, 19 patients were unchanged or worsened, and 1 patient was incompletely documented for pain on movement) [87].

In addition to these open-label trials, collagen hydrolysate has been studied in a prospective, randomized, double-blind, placebo-controlled clinical trial conducted by Adam [85]. Researchers recruited 81 patients with osteoarthritis of the knee or hip and used a complex crossover design to compare four different nutritional supplements that included collagen hydrolysate (10 g in the form of 20 capsules, each 500 mg, by mouth). They found that 81% of patients taking collagen hydrolysate achieved meaningful pain reduction compared with 23% of patients taking a control substance (egg albumin). In addition, 69% of patients taking collagen hydrolysate had a 50% or greater decrease in the consumption of analgesics compared with 35% of the patients taking egg albumin [85]. The author noted that the results from treatment with all nutritional supplements, including collagen hydrolysate, were significantly different from egg albumin, but he did not define statistical significance [85].

Another study of collagen hydrolysate by Moskowitz [86] was a prospective, randomized, double-blind, placebo-controlled clinical trial. The study included sites in Germany, the United Kingdom, and the United States and recruited 389 patients with knee osteoarthritis. Patients were randomly assigned to receive 10 g of collagen hydrolysate per day or placebo, by mouth, for 24 weeks. The primary outcome measures were the WOMAC pain score, function score, and patient global assessment. After 24 weeks of treatment, there were no statistically significant differences for the total study group for differences of mean score for pain. Moskowitz [86] reported, however, that one group of patients (the German patients, $n = 112$) experienced a statistically significant benefit from collagen hydrolysate in terms of pain reduction ($P = .016$) and functional improvement ($P = .007$), but not patient global evaluation ($P = .074$).

The benefits of collagen hydrolysate for patients with mild symptoms of osteoarthritis were examined in a randomized, placebo-controlled, double-blind study with 250 adults diagnosed with mild symptoms of osteoarthritis of the knee. A total of 190 patients completed the study (88 treatment and 102 placebo patients). Treatment consisted of oral administration of collagen hydrolysate (10 g/d) or placebo for 14 weeks. Isokinetic and isometric leg strength was assessed using a Biodex Multi-Joint System B2000 [89]. A 6-minute walk test and a 50-foot walk test were used to assess functional mobility, and joint pain, stiffness, and perceived functional mobility were assessed using the WOMAC Index, the Lequesne Index, and the Knee Pain Scale.

After 14 weeks of treatment, there were no statistically significant differences between the treatment groups for measures of pain, stiffness, mobility, or flexibility measurements. The collagen hydrolysate–treated group showed statistically significant improvement, however, in three out of six isokinetic leg strength measures (peak torque/body weight for extension at 60°/sec^{-1}, peak torque/body weight for flexion at 60°/sec^{-1}, and total work/body weight for extension at 60°/sec^{-1}; $P < .05$ compared with placebo for all three tests) [88]. The investigators stated the findings suggest that collagen hydrolysate may contribute to early changes in knee cartilage (M. Carpenter, personal communication, 2006), which is consistent with animal data [81].

SUMMARY

Osteoarthritis is a widespread condition that causes pain, disability, and decreased quality of life. Dietitians can play an important role in managing patients with osteoarthritis by supporting healthy eating habits, which should include the nutrients that support healthy joints. They also can encourage patients who are obese to reduce weight and increase activity levels.

Joints require many nutrients to stay healthy and to regenerate new tissue, including calcium, phosphorus, protein, vitamin C, vitamin D, vitamin E, and zinc. It also is important to include collagenous materials in the diet to maintain joint health, although many individuals may be cutting back on the amount of collagen in their diet. Joints are threatened further by overweight.

Joint disorders can result from many different causes, including stress to joints, poor dietary habits, injury or trauma, disease, obesity, aging, and congenital deformity. Regardless of the cause, there is no cure for joint disease. Treatment for joint disorders such as osteoarthritis focuses on reducing the pain and inflammation of affected joints, with the goal of maintaining mobility and maximizing quality of life.

Treatments for patients with osteoarthritis range from lifestyle changes, such as exercise, stretching, aerobic activities, and weight management, to dietary and nutritional interventions, including increasing levels of such nutrients as omega-3 fatty acids, vitamin C, and vitamin E. In addition, pharmacologic treatments, herbs, and nutritional supplements have been investigated for patients with osteoarthritis.

Drugs that have been used to manage symptoms of patients with osteoarthritis include NSAIDs, COX-2 inhibitors, and glucocorticoids. Herbal products include green tea extracts, SKI306X, and devil's claw. Nutritional supplements that have been studied in osteoarthritis patients include glucosamine and chondroitin sulfate, MSM, SAMe, and collagen hydrolysate. Research with these drugs and supplements has provided varying results about their efficacy in patients with osteoarthritis; additional research is needed to determine the optimal treatments for patients with this disorder.

References

[1] Clegg DO, Reda DJ, Harris CL, et al. Glucosamine, chondroitin sulfate, and the two in combination for painful knee osteoarthritis. N Engl J Med 2006;354:795–808.

[2] United States Senate Committee on Health E, Labor and Pensions, Subcommittee on Aging. Centers for Disease Control's role in combating the burden of arthritis. Washington, DC: Department of Health and Human Services; 2004.
[3] Cotran RS, Kumar V, Collins T, editors. Pathologic basis of disease. 6th edition. Philadelphia: Saunders; 1999.
[4] Resnick D. Common disorders of synovium-lined joints: pathogenesis, imaging abnormalities, and complications. AJR Am J Roentgenol 1988;151:1079–93.
[5] Young AA, Smith MM, Smith SM, et al. Regional assessment of articular cartilage gene expression and small proteoglycan metabolism in an animal model of osteoarthritis. Arthritis Res Ther 2005;7:R852–61.
[6] Brandt KD. Osteoarthritis. In: Braunwald E, Fauci AS, Kasper DL, et al, editors. Harrison's principles of internal medicine. 15th edition. New York: McGraw-Hill; 2001. p. 1987–94.
[7] Rosier RN, O'Keefe RJ. Autocrine regulation of articular cartilage. Instr Course Lect 1998;47:469–75.
[8] Baker CL Jr, Ferguson CM. Future treatment of osteoarthritis. Orthopedics 2005;28 (2 Suppl):s227–34.
[9] Trippel SB. Growth factor actions on articular cartilage. J Rheumatol 1995;43(Suppl):129–32.
[10] Poole AR. Cartilage in health and disease. In: McCarty DJ, Koopman WJ, editors. Arthritis and allied conditions: a textbook of rheumatology. Philadelphia: Lea & Febiger; 1993. p. 279–333.
[11] Rizzo R, Grandolfo M, Godeas C, et al. Calcium, sulfur, and zinc distribution in normal and arthritic articular equine cartilage: a synchrotron radiation-induced X-ray emission (SRIXE) study. J Exp Zool 1995;273:82–6.
[12] Clark AG, Rohrbaugh AL, Otterness I, et al. The effects of ascorbic acid on cartilage metabolism in guinea pig articular cartilage explants. Matrix Biol 2002;21:175–84.
[13] Wang Y, Prentice LF, Vitetta L, et al. The effect of nutritional supplements on osteoarthritis. Altern Med Rev 2004;9:275–96.
[14] Gerstenfeld LC, Kelly CM, Von Deck M, et al. Effect of 1,25-dihydroxyvitamin D3 on induction of chondrocyte maturation in culture: extracellular matrix gene expression and morphology. Endocrinology 1990;126:1599–609.
[15] White-O'Connor B, Sobal J. Nutrient intake and obesity in a multidisciplinary assessment of osteoarthritis. Clin Ther 1986;9(Suppl B):30–42.
[16] McAlindon TE, Felson DT, Zhang Y, et al. Relation of dietary intake and serum levels of vitamin D to progression of osteoarthritis of the knee among participants in the Framingham study. Ann Intern Med 1996;125:353–9.
[17] Tiku ML, Shah R, Allison GT. Evidence linking chondrocyte lipid peroxidation to cartilage matrix protein degradation: possible role in cartilage aging and the pathogenesis of osteoarthritis. J Biol Chem 2000;275:20069–76.
[18] Kaiki G, Tsuji H, Yonezawa T, et al. Osteoarthrosis induced by intra-articular hydrogen peroxide injection and running load. J Orthop Res 1990;8:731–40.
[19] Kowsari B, Finnie SK, Carter RL, et al. Assessment of the diet of patients with rheumatoid arthritis and osteoarthritis. J Am Diet Assoc 1983;82:657–9.
[20] Grennan DM, Knudson JM, Dunckley J, et al. Serum copper and zinc in rheumatoid arthritis and osteoarthritis. N Z Med J 1980;91:47–50.
[21] Meachin G, Brooks G. The pathology of osteoarthritis. In: Moskowitz RW, Howell DS, Goldberg VM, et al, editors. Osteoarthritis: diagnosis and management. Philadelphia: Saunders; 1984. p. 29–42.
[22] Howell DS. Pathogenesis of osteoarthritis. Am J Med 1986;80(4B):24–8.
[23] Adams ME. Pathogenesis of osteoarthritis. In: Hadler NM, editor. Clinical concepts in regional musculoskeletal illness. Orlando (FL): Grune & Stratton; 1987. p. 137–67.
[24] Hamerman D. The biology of osteoarthritis. N Engl J Med 1989;320:1322–30.
[25] Spector TD. The fat on the joint: osteoarthritis and obesity. J Rheumatol 1990;17:283–4.

[26] Felson DT, Anderson JJ, Naimark A, et al. Obesity and knee osteoarthritis. The Framingham Study. Ann Intern Med 1988;109:18–24.
[27] Coggon D, Reading I, Croft P, et al. Knee osteoarthritis and obesity. Int J Obes Relat Metab Disord 2001;25:622–7.
[28] Carman WJ, Sowers M, Hawthorne VM, et al. Obesity as a risk factor for osteoarthritis of the hand and wrist: a prospective study. Am J Epidemiol 1994;139:119–29.
[29] Cicuttini FM, Baker JR, Spector TD. The association of obesity with osteoarthritis of the hand and knee in women: a twin study. J Rheumatol 1996;23:1221–6.
[30] Haara MM, Manninen P, Kroger H, et al. Osteoarthritis of finger joints in Finns aged 30 or over: prevalence, determinants, and association with mortality. Ann Rheum Dis 2003;62: 151–8.
[31] Wilhelmi G. [Potential influence of nutrition with supplements on healthy and arthritic joints. II. Nutritional quantity, supplements, contamination]. Z Rheumatol 1993;52:191–200.
[32] Exercise prescription for older adults with osteoarthritis pain: consensus practice recommendations. A supplement to the AGS Clinical Practice Guidelines on the management of chronic pain in older adults. J Am Geriatr Soc 2001;49:808–23.
[33] O'Reilly SC, Muir KR, Doherty M. Effectiveness of home exercise on pain and disability from osteoarthritis of the knee: a randomised controlled trial. Ann Rheum Dis 1999; 58:15–9.
[34] Marks R. The effect of isometric quadriceps strength training in mid-range for osteoarthritis of the knee. Arthritis Care Res 1993;6:52–6.
[35] Fisher NM, Pendergast DR, Gresham GE, et al. Muscle rehabilitation: its effect on muscular and functional performance of patients with knee osteoarthritis. Arch Phys Med Rehabil 1991;72:367–74.
[36] Deyle GD, Henderson NE, Matekel RL, et al. Effectiveness of manual physical therapy and exercise in osteoarthritis of the knee: a randomized, controlled trial. Ann Intern Med 2000; 132:173–81.
[37] Thomas KS, Muir KR, Doherty M, et al. Home based exercise programme for knee pain and knee osteoarthritis: randomised controlled trial. BMJ 2002;325:752.
[38] Schwartz ER, Leveille CR, Stevens JW, et al. Proteoglycan structure and metabolism in normal and osteoarthritic cartilage of guinea pigs. Arthritis Rheum 1981;24:1528–39.
[39] Schwartz ER, Oh WH, Leveille CR. Experimentally induced osteoarthritis in guinea pigs: metabolic responses in articular cartilage to developing pathology. Arthritis Rheum 1981; 24:1345–55.
[40] McAlindon TE, Jacques P, Zhang Y, et al. Do antioxidant micronutrients protect against the development and progression of knee osteoarthritis? Arthritis Rheum 1996;39: 648–56.
[41] Jensen NH. [Reduced pain from osteoarthritis in hip joint or knee joint during treatment with calcium ascorbate: a randomized, placebo-controlled cross-over trial in general practice]. Ugeskr Laeger 2003;165:2563–6.
[42] Blankenhorn G. [Clinical effectiveness of Spondyvit (vitamin E) in activated arthroses: a multicenter placebo-controlled double-blind study]. Z Orthop Ihre Grenzgeb 1986;124: 340–3.
[43] Machtey I, Ouaknine L. Tocopherol in osteoarthritis: a controlled pilot study. J Am Geriatr Soc 1978;26:328–30.
[44] Scherak O, Kolarz G, Schodl C, et al. [High dosage vitamin E therapy in patients with activated arthrosis]. Z Rheumatol 1990;49:369–73.
[45] Brand C, Snaddon J, Bailey M, et al. Vitamin E is ineffective for symptomatic relief of knee osteoarthritis: a six month double blind, randomised, placebo controlled study. Ann Rheum Dis 2001;60:946–9.
[46] Wluka AE, Stuckey S, Brand C, et al. Supplementary vitamin E does not affect the loss of cartilage volume in knee osteoarthritis: a 2 year double blind randomized placebo controlled study. J Rheumatol 2002;29:2585–91.

[47] Dougados M. Why and how to use NSAIDs in osteoarthritis. J Cardiovasc Pharmacol 2006;47(Suppl 1):S49–54.

[48] Brandt KD. Should nonsteroidal anti-inflammatory drugs be used to treat osteoarthritis? Rheum Dis Clin N Am 1993;19:29–44.

[49] Mitchell JA, Akarasereenont P, Thiemermann C, et al. Selectivity of nonsteroidal antiinflammatory drugs as inhibitors of constitutive and inducible cyclooxygenase. Proc Natl Acad Sci U S A 1993;90:11693–7.

[50] Silverstein FE, Faich G, Goldstein JL, et al. Gastrointestinal toxicity with celecoxib vs nonsteroidal anti-inflammatory drugs for osteoarthritis and rheumatoid arthritis: the CLASS study: a randomized controlled trial. Celecoxib Long-term Arthritis Safety Study. JAMA 2000;284:1247–55.

[51] Bombardier C, Laine L, Reicin A, et al. Comparison of upper gastrointestinal toxicity of rofecoxib and naproxen in patients with rheumatoid arthritis. VIGOR Study Group. N Engl J Med 2000;343:1520–8.

[52] Levesque LE, Brophy JM, Zhang B. Time variations in the risk of myocardial infarction among elderly users of COX-2 inhibitors. Can Med Assoc J 2006;174:1563–9.

[53] Towheed TE, Hochberg MC. A systematic review of randomized controlled trials of pharmacological therapy in osteoarthritis of the knee, with an emphasis on trial methodology. Semin Arthritis Rheum 1997;26:755–70.

[54] Raynauld JP, Buckland-Wright C, Ward R, et al. Safety and efficacy of long-term intraarticular steroid injections in osteoarthritis of the knee: a randomized, double-blind, placebo-controlled trial. Arthritis Rheum 2003;48:370–7.

[55] Recommendations for the medical management of osteoarthritis of the hip and knee: 2000 update. American College of Rheumatology Subcommittee on Osteoarthritis Guidelines. Arthritis Rheum 2000;43:1905–15.

[56] Pendleton A, Arden N, Dougados M, et al. EULAR recommendations for the management of knee osteoarthritis: report of a task force of the Standing Committee for International Clinical Studies Including Therapeutic Trials (ESCISIT). Ann Rheum Dis 2000;59:936–44.

[57] Gossec L, Dougados M. Intra-articular treatments in osteoarthritis: from the symptomatic to the structure modifying. Ann Rheum Dis 2004;63:478–82.

[58] Curtis CL, Harwood JL, Dent CM, et al. Biological basis for the benefit of nutraceutical supplementation in arthritis. Drug Discov Today 2004;9:165–72.

[59] Haqqi TM, Anthony DD, Gupta S, et al. Prevention of collagen-induced arthritis in mice by a polyphenolic fraction from green tea. Proc Natl Acad Sci U S A 1999;96:4524–9.

[60] Adcocks C, Collin P, Buttle DJ. Catechins from green tea (*Camellia sinensis*) inhibit bovine and human cartilage proteoglycan and type II collagen degradation in vitro. J Nutr 2002;132:341–6.

[61] Singh R, Ahmed S, Islam N, et al. Epigallocatechin-3-gallate inhibits interleukin-1beta-induced expression of nitric oxide synthase and production of nitric oxide in human chondrocytes: suppression of nuclear factor kappaB activation by degradation of the inhibitor of nuclear factor kappaB. Arthritis Rheum 2002;46:2079–86.

[62] Tao X, Younger J, Fan FZ, et al. Benefit of an extract of Tripterygium Wilfordii Hook F in patients with rheumatoid arthritis: a double-blind, placebo-controlled study. Arthritis Rheum 2002;46:1735–43.

[63] Choi JH, Choi JH, Kim DY, et al. Effects of SKI 306X, a new herbal agent, on proteoglycan degradation in cartilage explant culture and collagenase-induced rabbit osteoarthritis model. Osteoarthritis Cartilage 2002;6:471–8.

[64] Chrubasik S, Pollak S, Black A. Effectiveness of devil's claw for osteoarthritis. Rheumatology (Oxford) 2002;41:1332–3; author reply 1333.

[65] Gagnier JJ, Chrubasik S, Manheimer E. *Harpgophytum procumbens* for osteoarthritis and low back pain: a systematic review. BMC Complement Altern Med 2004;4:13.

[66] Annual nutrition industry overview. Nutrition Business J 2005;10:6–7.

[67] Kelly GS. The role of glucosamine sulfate and chondroitin sulfates in the treatment of degenerative joint disease. Altern Med Rev 1998;3:27–39.
[68] Zhu X, Cai J, Yang J, et al. Determination of glucosamine in impure chitin samples by high-performance liquid chromatography. Carbohydr Res 2005;340:1732–8.
[69] Tiraloche G, Girard C, Chouinard L, et al. Effect of oral glucosamine on cartilage degradation in a rabbit model of osteoarthritis. Arthritis Rheum 2005;52:1118–28.
[70] Karzel K, Lee KJ. [Effect of hexosamine derivatives on mesenchymal metabolic processes of in vitro cultured fetal bone explants]. Z Rheumatol 1982;41:212–8.
[71] Setnikar I, Cereda R, Pacini MA, et al. Antireactive properties of glucosamine sulfate. Arzneimittelforschung 1991;41:157–61.
[72] Michel BA, Stucki G, Frey D, et al. Chondroitins 4 and 6 sulfate in osteoarthritis of the knee: a randomized, controlled trial. Arthritis Rheum 2005;52:779–86.
[73] Cibere J, Thorne A, Kopec JA, et al. Glucosamine sulfate and cartilage type II collagen degradation in patients with knee osteoarthritis: randomized discontinuation trial results employing biomarkers. J Rheumatol 2005;32:896–902.
[74] McAlindon TE, LaValley MP, Gulin JP, et al. Glucosamine and chondroitin for treatment of osteoarthritis: a systematic quality assessment and meta-analysis. JAMA 2000;283:1469–75.
[75] Kim LS, Axelrod LJ, Howard P, et al. Efficacy of methylsulfonylmethane (MSM) in osteoarthritis pain of the knee: a pilot clinical trial. Osteoarthritis Cartilage 2006;14:286–94.
[76] Najm WI, Reinsch S, Hoehler F, et al. S-adenosyl methionine (SAMe) versus celecoxib for the treatment of osteoarthritis symptoms: a double-blind cross-over trial [ISRCTN36233495]. BMC Musculoskelet Disord 2004;5:6.
[77] Harmand MF, Vilamitjana J, Maloche E, et al. Effects of S-adenosylmethionine on human articular chondrocyte differentiation: an in vitro study. Am J Med 1987;83:48–54.
[78] Katzenstein PL, Malemud CJ, Pathria MN, et al. Early-onset primary osteoarthritis and mild chondrodysplasia: radiographic and pathologic studies with an analysis of cartilage proteoglycans. Arthritis Rheum 1990;33:674–84.
[79] Knowlton RG, Katzenstein PL, Moskowitz RW, et al. Genetic linkage of a polymorphism in the type II procollagen gene (COL2A1) to primary osteoarthritis associated with mild chondrodysplasia. N Engl J Med 1990;322:526–30.
[80] Lohmann M. Untersuchungen zur Bedeutung von Gelatine als Proteinbestandteil. Inauguraldissertation; Agrarwissenschaftliche Fakultät, Universität Kiel; 1994.
[81] Oesser S, Adam M, Babel W, et al. Oral administration of (14)C labeled gelatin hydrolysate leads to an accumulation of radioactivity in cartilage of mice (C57/BL). J Nutr 1999;129:1891–5.
[82] Krug E. Zur unterstützenden Therapie bei Osteo- und Chondropathien. Zeitschrift für Erfahrungsheikunde 1979;11:930–8.
[83] Götz B. Gut genährter Knorpel knirscht nicht mehr. Arztl Prax 1982;92:3130–4.
[84] Oberschelp U. Individuelle Arthrosetherapie ist möglich. Therapiewoche 1985;44:5094–7.
[85] Adam M. Welche Wirkung haben Gelatinepräparate? Therapie der Osteoarthrose. Therapiewoche 1991;41:2456–61.
[86] Moskowitz RW. Role of collagen hydrolysate in bone and joint disease. Semin Arthritis Rheum 2000;30:87–99.
[87] Flechsenhar K, Alf D. Ergebnisse einer Anwendungsbeobachtung zu Kollagen-Hydrolysat CH-Alpha. Orthopaedische Praxis 2005;9:486–94.
[88] Zuckley L, Angelopoulou K, Carpenter M, et al. Collagen hydrolysate improves joint function in adults with mild symptoms of osteoarthritis of the knee. Presented at 51st Annual American College of Sports Medicine. Indianapolis (IN), June 2–4, 2004.
[89] Zuckley L, Angelopoulou K, Carpenter MR, et al. Collagen hydrolysate improves joint function in adults with mild symptoms of osteoarthritis of the knee. Med Sci Sports Exerc 2004;36(Suppl):S153–4.

ELSEVIER
SAUNDERS

Clin Sports Med 26 (2007) 119–130

CLINICS IN SPORTS MEDICINE

Micronutrient Requirements for Athletes

Stella Lucia Volpe, PhD, RD, LDN

Division of Biobehavioral and Health Sciences, School of Nursing, University of Pennsylvania, Nursing Education Building, 420 Guardian Drive, Philadelphia, PA 19104-6096, USA

Vitamins and minerals are necessary for many metabolic processes in the body and are important in supporting growth and development [1]. Vitamins and minerals also are required in numerous reactions involved with exercise and physical activity, including energy, carbohydrate, fat and protein metabolism, oxygen transfer and delivery, and tissue repair [1]. The vitamin and mineral needs of athletes have always been a topic of discussion. Some researchers state that athletes require more vitamins and minerals than their sedentary counterparts, whereas other researchers do not report greater micronutrient requirements. The intensity, duration, and frequency of the sport/workout and the overall energy and nutrient intakes of the individual all have an impact on whether or not micronutrients are required in greater amounts [1–3]. This article evaluates the vitamin and mineral needs of athletes.

DIETARY REFERENCE INTAKES

The Dietary Reference Intakes (DRI) for all known vitamins and essential minerals for healthy individuals living in the United States were updated between 1997 and 2005 [4–8]. Adequate Intake (AI), Recommended Dietary Allowance (RDA), Estimated Average Requirement (EAR), and Tolerable Upper Intake Level (UL) all are under the DRI heading. The RDA is the dietary intake level that is sufficient for approximately 98% of healthy individuals living in the United States. The AI is a projected value that is used when the RDA cannot be established. The EAR is a value used to estimate the nutrient requirements of half of the healthy individuals in a group [8]. The UL is the maximum quantity of a nutrient most individuals can consume without resulting in adverse side effects [8]. The DRIs for all nutrients may be found at the following website: http://www.iom.edu/Object.File/Master/21/372/0.pdf.

In most cases, if energy intakes are sufficient, the micronutrient requirements of athletes are similar to healthy, fairly active individuals; using the DRI for evaluating nutrient needs would be suitable. Some athletes may have greater requirements, however, as a result of disproportionate losses of nutrients in

E-mail address: svolpe@nursing.upenn.edu

0278-5919/07/$ – see front matter
doi:10.1016/j.csm.2006.11.009

© 2007 Elsevier Inc. All rights reserved.

sweat and urine. For these athletes, supplementation may need to be considered on an individual basis. Many athletes supplement with vitamins, minerals, and ergogenic aids on their own. The UL provides guidelines to athletes who supplement, which should prevent negative effects from occurring owing to oversupplementation.

IMPORTANCE OF ACCURATE DIETARY INTAKE ASSESSMENT

Although this article focuses on micronutrients, a total evaluation of an athlete's energy intake is necessary because even if an athlete is consuming the correct amount of micronutrients (especially if he or she is supplementing with a vitamin-mineral supplement), if energy requirements are not being met, athletic performance still would be suboptimal. Clark and colleagues [9] examined the preseason and postseason intakes of macronutrients and micronutrients in division I female soccer players. They reported that despite meeting total energy requirements (carbohydrate needs were not met), vitamin E, folate, copper, and magnesium intakes were suboptimal (<75% of the DRI).

The evaluation of an athlete's diet must be conducted properly to ensure accuracy [10]. It is common for athletes (and nonathletes) to underreport their dietary intake. Consequently, it is imperative that athletes are taught how to estimate accurately portion sizes and fluid intake, the amount and frequency of snacking, any weight management practices they may perform, and changes in their food patterns during seasons and off-seasons [10].

MICRONUTRIENT INTAKE AND NUTRITION STATUS AMONG ATHLETES

Dietary Intake Assessment and Nutritional Status in Male Athletes

Assessing dietary intake among any individual is difficult and is often criticized because of the inherent lack of accuracy. Nonetheless, dietary records are still the best method presently available to estimate dietary intake. Although dietary records often provide information about intake at a particular point in time, longer term studies can help to provide a more accurate assessment of dietary intake, even if one point in time is assessed per year. Leblanc and coworkers [11] analyzed the diets of French male athletes training at the National Training Centre in Clairefontaine. There were 180 athletes, 13 to 16 years old, who participated in this 3-year dietary survey. Despite the long-term nature of this study, calcium and iron were the only micronutrients evaluated. Each year, a 5-day food record was collected from these athletes. Leblanc and coworkers [11] reported insufficient energy intake for all athletes. They also reported that calcium intake was below recommendations during the first year, whereas iron intake was sufficient; however, calcium and iron intakes significantly improved ($P<.05$) over the 3-year period [11]. The researchers stated that the increase in calcium and iron intake may have been a result of a physiologic adjustment to growth or to the positive effects of the nutrition courses provided during their stay at the Centre [11]. Rico-Sanz and colleagues [12] also reported lower than recommended intakes of calcium in eight male soccer players (average age 17 years) who were part of the Puerto Rican Olympic soccer team, despite an adequate energy intake.

Iglesias-Gutierrez and associates [13] evaluated the dietary intake and nutritional status of adolescent Spanish soccer players of similar age to those studied by Leblanc and coworkers [11] (14–16 years old; $n = 33$). The soccer players consumed an adequate amount of iron; however, 48% of these athletes were iron deficient (without anemia). These results suggest that even with adequate intakes of micronutrients, the impact of training may require greater amounts of certain micronutrients. A nutrition intervention, including education and monitoring transient and long-term micronutrient changes (intake and blood values), is required to make definitive recommendations, however [13,14]. It has been suggested that nutrition education be provided to athletes at an early age and continued throughout adolescence, not only to optimize athletic performance, but also to promote healthy dietary practices throughout the life span [14].

In a more recent study, Paschoal and Amancio [15] examined the dietary intake and nutritional status of eight Brazilian elite male swimmers, 18 to 21 years old. Four-day dietary records indicated adequate energy and micronutrient intake, with the exception of calcium, for which only four of the athletes consumed the recommended amount. The biochemical indices of nutritional status all were within normal limits for the micronutrients. These researchers also reported that 62.5% and 25% of the swimmers consumed amino acid and antioxidant supplements. Similar to other researchers, Paschoal and Amancio [15] strongly recommended nutrition education for balanced dietary intake and education about supplementation.

Rankinen and associates [16] also evaluated the dietary intake and nutritional status of athletes (Finnish elite male ski jumpers) ($n = 21$), but compared them with age-matched controls ($n = 20$). Dietary intake was assessed via 4-day dietary records. There were no differences between groups in age and height, although the ski jumpers had a lower mean body weight and percent body fat (assessed via dual-energy x-ray absorptiometry). Energy intake was significantly lower ($P = .001$) in the ski jumpers compared with the control participants. Despite this difference in energy intake, thiamine, riboflavin, folate, vitamin C, calcium, and iron intakes were similar between groups; however, vitamins D and E, zinc, and magnesium were significantly lower in the ski jumpers compared with the controls. Although the ski jumpers had significantly lower intakes of these micronutrients, their biochemical markers of nutritional status were within normal limits. Although nutritional status was within normal limits, the cross-sectional nature of this and many other studies to determine nutritional status among athletes may not accurately capture deficiencies that could be occurring over time. Blood (plasma or serum) concentrations of micronutrients are not always the best measure of status.

Dietary Intake Assessment and Nutritional Status in Female Athletes

There seems to be more research on the dietary intake of female athletes than male athletes, probably because of a higher prevalence of disordered eating among women, especially in sports that require a specific body weight to compete or in sports that also highly value esthetics. Ziegler and colleagues [17] evaluated 18 female competitive figure skaters, 14 to 16 years old, during preseason, the competitive season, and off-season using 3-day dietary records. Energy intake was below energy needs, although energy intake did not differ significantly over the three seasons. Nonetheless, throughout the competitive season, 78%, 50%, and 44% of the skaters had intakes less than 67% of the RDA for folate, iron, and calcium. The biochemical indicators of nutritional status were within normal limits, although long-term assessments are required to evaluate the impact of the less-than-adequate intake of the aforementioned nutrients. Ziegler and colleagues [17] emphasized the need for nutrition education among these athletes, especially throughout their competitive season.

Hassapidou and Manstrantoni [18] compared the dietary intake of elite Greek female athletes in four different sports (volleyball, middle distance running, ballet dancing, and swimming) with a nonathletic control group. They evaluated dietary intake using 7-day weighed dietary records over two seasons, the training season and the competitive season. The investigators reported a lower than recommended intake of iron in the athletic and nonathletic groups, but a higher than recommended intake of vitamin C in all participants, which they stated was "characteristic of the population of the Mediterranean countries" [18]. Although micronutrient intakes did not differ between athletes and nonathletes, biochemical indices to assess status were not conducted. An additional study on dietary intake conducted in female Greek athletes (volleyball players) found that these adolescent athletes did not consume recommended intakes for calcium, iron, folate, magnesium, zinc, vitamin A, and the B vitamins [19]. Neither of these groups of researchers evaluated nutritional status; nevertheless, the lower than recommended intake could lead to less than optimal performance and growth (in the adolescent athletes).

Beals [20] conducted a more complete study on 23 nationally ranked female adolescent volleyball players. Nutrient intake was assessed using 3-day weighed food records. Iron, vitamins C and B_{12}, and folate status were determined through blood samples. Beals [20] found that these athletes consumed fewer calories than they expended (energy intake $= 2248 \pm 414$ kcal/d, energy expenditure $= 2815$ kcal/d). They also consumed less than the recommended intakes for folate, B-complex vitamins, vitamin C, iron, calcium, magnesium, and zinc. With respect to their nutritional status, three of the athletes had iron deficiency anemia, one athlete had a marginal vitamin B_{12} status, and four athletes had marginal vitamin C status. Beals [20] also reported a high percentage of athletes who had past or present menstrual disorders (amenorrhea, oligomenorrhea, or irregular menstrual cycles). The combination of low energy and micronutrient intake and menstrual irregularities shows the need for long-term studies evaluating dietary intake and nutritional status among athletes of all levels and ages.

In another comprehensive study, Kim and coworkers [21] compared the nutritional intake, iron status, and immunologic patterns of Korean female Judo athletes to control participants. Three-day dietary records were used to evaluate intake. In general, vitamin and mineral intakes were within recommendations; however, calcium and iron intakes were less than 100% of the recommendations, whereas intakes of phosphorus, thiamine, and riboflavin were greater in athletes compared with controls. None of the participants were iron deficient; however, iron, thiamine, and niacin intakes were positively associated with the immunologic variables measured. Although more research is required on the dietary intake and nutritional status of all athletes, further investigation is needed in the area of specific vitamins and minerals with immunologic function in athletes, especially endurance athletes [21].

Athletes of all levels of competition can be negatively affected by poor dietary intake. Heptathletes are so varied in their training and competition, by the mere nature of their sport, that they may be at greater risk for nutritional deficiencies. Mullins and coworkers [22] assessed the dietary intake (using 4-day dietary records) and nutritional status of 19 female heptathletes, 26 ± 3 years of age, during their training season. These athletes consumed more than 67% of the recommended intakes for all nutrients, with the exception of vitamin E, despite the fact that more than 50% of this group took vitamin supplements. Biochemical markers indicated normal iron status. The cross-sectional nature of this study, similar to some of the previously discussed studies, may not accurately reflect dietary intake and nutritional status.

In two separate studies, Gropper and colleagues [23,24] evaluated the copper and iron intake and status of 70 female collegiate athletes (18–25 years old) from across different sports. Depending on the sport, copper intake ranged from 41% to 118% of the recommended intakes. Of the athletes, 41% did not consume two thirds of the RDA for copper. Serum copper and ceruloplasmin concentrations were within normal limits for all athletes. With respect to iron intake and status, 25% of the athletes did not consume two thirds of the RDA for iron, and these athletes displayed suboptimal serum ferritin, iron, or transferring saturation concentrations [24]. Athletes whose serum ferritin concentration was 15 μg/L or less also displayed serum iron concentrations of less than 60 μg/dL and transferrin saturation of less than 16% (both below normal). Despite the fact that these were athletes from different sports, and iron deficiency was not apparent, iron depletion was present in many of these athletes across different sports and different ages. Certain studies have suggested that iron-depleted women have decreased maximal oxygen consumption ($V\text{O}_2$max) as a result of decreased iron storage [25]. Some studies have observed alterations in metabolic rate, thyroid hormone status, and thermoregulation with iron depletion and iron deficiency anemia [26–29], although some researchers have not observed these alterations [30]. Mild iron deficiency anemia also has been shown to affect psychomotor development, intellectual performance, and immune function negatively [31,32]. The fact the iron deficiency anemia is one of the most common nutritional deficiencies throughout the world, especially in women, further emphasizes the need for proper nutrition education and intake among female athletes.

The previously discussed studies all have been cross-sectional in nature, which provides a snapshot of the athletes' intake and status, but do not allow for further interpretation. Petersen and associates [33] evaluated 18 female collegiate swimmers and 6 female collegiate divers preseason and after 16 weeks of training. There were no changes in energy intake over time; however, the athletes significantly improved their dietary quality as evidenced by increases in iron, vitamin C, and vitamin B_6 intake. The investigators also reported improved iron status in these athletes, with increases in hemoglobin and hematocrit, with a subsequent decrease in serum transferrin receptors. Clark and coworkers [9] assessed dietary intake in female collegiate soccer players preseason to postseason and reported marginal intakes (<75% of the DRI) for vitamin E, folate, copper, and magnesium, with no improvements over the season as Petersen and associates [33] reported. Although these studies evaluated preseason to postseason dietary intake or nutritional status, research examining intake over a longer period is needed to assess fully any impact of poor dietary intake on nutritional status and performance.

Dietary Intake Assessment and Nutritional Status in Special Populations of Female Athletes

Female athletes may be more restrictive in their dietary intake than male athletes, placing them at greater risk for nutritional deficiencies and impaired performance and health. Beals and Manore [34] evaluated the diet and nutritional status of female athletes with subclinical eating disorders ($n = 24$), compared with those of controls ($n = 24$). The group with subclinical eating disorders had significantly lower energy intake than the control group (1989 kcal/d versus 2300 kcal/d; $P = .004$); however, energy expenditure did not differ between groups. Average micronutrient intake and iron, zinc, magnesium, vitamin B_{12}, and folate status did not differ between groups (and were within normal limits). Athletes in both groups used vitamin-mineral supplements, which likely improved nutritional status.

Aside from disordered eating, many female athletes are vegetarians for various reasons, which also could affect nutritional intake and status. Janelle and Barr [35] compared the nutrient intakes of vegetarian ($n = 23$) and nonvegetarian ($n = 22$) athletes, 20 to 40 years old, using 3-day dietary records. The vegetarian athletes had lower intakes of riboflavin, niacin, vitamin B_{12}, zinc, and sodium intakes, while consuming higher intakes of folate, vitamin C, and copper compared with the nonvegetarians. Within the subgroup of the vegetarians, vegans consumed lower calcium and vitamin B_{12} compared with lactovegetarians. Despite the health-conscious nature of many vegetarians, dietary intake still may be inadequate and is definitely not the same among subgroups of vegetarians. Vegetarian athletes may need more information on proper nutritional intake to ensure adequate energy and micronutrient intake for optimal performance and health.

Dietary Intake Assessment and Nutritional Status in Female and Male Athletes

Numerous researchers evaluated the dietary intake of female and male athletes from similar sports. These studies can help shed some light on gender differences within the same sports. Although the total nutrient intake of athletes is important, evaluating the diversity of athletes' meals and snacks in providing nutrients is also important. Ziegler and colleagues [36] evaluated the contribution of breakfast, lunch, dinner, and snacks on the macronutrient and micronutrient intake of 46 male and 48 female elite figure skaters who participated in the 1999 US National Figure Skating Championships. Three-day dietary records were used to assess dietary intake. With respect to micronutrient intake, they reported that breakfast was the main source of dietary folate (36%), whereas breakfast and dinner were the main sources of iron (29% and 27%) and calcium (32% and 29%). Ziegler and colleagues [36] concluded that these figure skaters needed to be educated about the benefits of consuming breakfast and about consuming a variety of foods throughout the day to maintain proper energy and micronutrient intake.

A larger study of the National Figure Skating Championship competitors was conducted in which 4-day diet records and fasting blood samples and anthropometric variables were assessed 2 months after the National Championships [37]. Forty-one figure skaters 11 to 18 years old participated in this study. The researchers compared their intakes with the Third National Health and Nutrition Examination Survey (NHANES III) and recommended intakes. Ziegler and colleagues [37] reported that the mean intakes for vitamins were greater than required intakes except for vitamins D and E. In addition, compared with NHANES III, the figure skaters consumed lower amounts of vitamins B_{12} and E, but greater amounts of vitamin C and thiamine (female skaters only). Male and female figure skaters consumed lower amounts of magnesium and zinc compared with recommended intakes. Male figure skaters also consumed lower amounts of iodine, whereas female figure skaters consumed lower amounts of magnesium, zinc, calcium, iron, and phosphorus compared with recommended intakes. Although biochemical indices of nutritional status were within the normal range, electrolyte concentrations indicated dehydration. Ziegler and colleagues [37] emphasized the need for dietary interventions and nutrition education for these athletes to lead to optimal performance and health.

In a more recent study from the same group of researchers, Jonnalagadda and colleagues [38] assessed the food preferences and nutrient intakes of elite male ($n = 23$) and female ($n = 26$) figure skaters using 3-day dietary records. They reported that male figure skaters had a higher preference for grains, meat, dairy, fats, fruit, and sweets, whereas female figure skaters had a higher preference for fruits and grains. Total energy intake and vitamins E and D, magnesium, and potassium intake were less than two thirds of the recommended intake for males and females. Female skaters also consumed less than two thirds of the recommended intakes for folate, pantothenic acid, calcium, and phosphorus. The researchers did not assess biochemical indices of these athletes; nutritional status could not be determined. Regardless, decreased intakes, combined with intense training, can lead to impaired performance and health.

Constantini and associates [39] assessed the iron status of Israeli male and female gymnasts 12 to 18 years old compared with summers, tennis players, and table tennis players. They all trained for about 25 hours per week, lived in the same national center for gifted athletes, and ate in the same dining room. Hemoglobin concentrations were less than 14 g/dL in 45% of the male gymnasts compared with only 25% of the nongymnasts and less than 13 g/dL in 25% of premenarcheal female gymnasts compared with 15% of nongymnasts. Iron depletion (serum ferritin levels <20 ng/mL) was observed in 36% of the male gymnasts and 30% of the female gymnasts. The prevalence of iron deficiency and depletion in the gymnasts compared with the other athletes was much greater and may be due to the pressures of maintaining a low body weight, even in males. Dubnov and Constantini [40] reported similar high rates of iron depletion and iron deficiency, however, in 103 male and female national basketball players. They reported that 15% of males and 25% of females were iron depleted, whereas 18% of males and 38% of females were iron deficient. These researchers recommend iron screening and nutritional counseling for athletes.

SUPPLEMENTATION AND ATHLETIC PERFORMANCE

Based on the aforementioned review, it seems that some athletes may need to supplement as a result of inadequate dietary intake or impaired nutritional status. Does supplementation improve performance, however? Tsalis and colleagues [41] evaluated whether the iron status of healthy adolescent swimmers was altered during a 6-month training season, and if increased daily iron intake (via supplement or food) would affect iron status or performance. Twenty-one male and 21 female Greek swimmers 12 to 17 years old were separated into three groups: (1) Group A received an iron supplement of 47 mg/d, (2) group B followed a diet high in iron (providing about 26 mg/d), and (3) group C served as the control group. Data were collected at baseline and at the end of three training phases. The investigators found significant variations in iron status during the training season; however, they did not find significant differences in iron status or performance among the three groups, which could have been due to the fact that these athletes were neither iron depleted nor iron deficient. Vasankari and associates [42] found no improvement in exercise-induced oxidative stress in Finnish runners who were supplemented with vitamin C. Although Bryant and colleagues [43] reported diminished membrane damage with 400 IU/d of vitamin E in trained cyclists (22.3 $\pm$ 2 years old, who participated in four separate supplementation trials–placebo, 1 g/d of vitamin C, 400 IU/d of vitamin E, or 1 g/d of vitamin C plus 200 IU/d of vitamin E), 1 g/d of vitamin C promoted cellular damage. Neither vitamin E nor vitamin C (alone or taken together) improved exercise performance.

Although these particular researchers did not find a positive effect on nutritional status or performance with supplementation, the nutritional status of the athletes is probably the key factor in why these trials were not as effective. It would seem that athletes who were deficient in particular micronutrients would benefit the most from supplementation, in terms of nutritional status and athletic performance. Conversely, with respect to vitamin C, Peake [44] stated,

"... it remains unclear if regular exercise increases the metabolism of vitamin C. However, the similar dietary intakes and responses to supplementation between athletes and non-athletes suggest that regular exercise does not increase the requirement for vitamin C in athletes."

LIMITATIONS IN RESEARCH

Although a great deal of research has been conducted on vitamins and minerals and athletes, more research is required. In addition, the research that has been published has limitations, including, but not limited to, the following: (1) small sample sizes; (2) mostly conducted in female athletes; (3) variations in type of sport studied; (4) variations in levels of training and fitness of athletes studied; (5) deficient in solid longitudinal data; (6) variations in methodology or study design (many have been cross-sectional); (7) differences in the types and amounts of supplementation used; and (8) some studies use a combination of vitamin and mineral supplements, making it difficult to ascertain the effects of one particular vitamin or mineral.

GENERAL RECOMMENDATIONS

Based on this review, athletes seem to consume inadequate amounts of many micronutrients (and energy); however, not all athletes have impaired nutritional status, which could be a result of study design and not their true status. Maughan [45] stated it well in his review, "When talented, motivated and highly trained athletes meet for competition the margin between victory and defeat is usually small. When everything else is equal, nutrition can make the difference between winning and losing." Economos and associates [46] published a review article in which they reviewed 22 research studies on the nutritional intake of athletes. Based on their review, they recommend an energy intake of greater than 50 kcal/kg/d for male athletes who train for more than 90 min/d and 45 to 50 kcal/kg/d for female athletes who train for more than 90 min/d. They also recommend that athletes who consume low-energy diets focus on adequate intakes of iron, calcium, magnesium, zinc, and vitamin B_{12}. "There is no special food that will help elite athletes perform better; the most important aspect of the diet of elite athletes is that it follows the basic guidelines for healthy eating" [46]. Athletes should work with a registered dietitian with expertise in sports nutrition to establish his or her nutritional and performance goals–goals that will lead to consistent eating and training, leading to improved performance [45]. With respect to micronutrients, it seems that if energy intake is sufficient, balanced, and varied, and nutritional status is within normal limits, vitamin-mineral supplementation is not warranted [45,47]. Supplementation may be warranted for athletes who restrict energy intake, participate in sports with weight restrictions, or limit certain foods and food groups [47].

SUMMARY

The micronutrient intake and status of athletes has been assessed in numerous researcher studies; however, limitations exist in many of these studies, owing to the cross-sectional nature of the study design. From the published data, however, it seems that athletes who consume adequate energy and micronutrients would not benefit from supplementation. Longitudinal research is required (including supplementation studies) to follow athletes over time and evaluate dietary intake, nutritional status, and effects of performance properly.

References

[1] Wardlaw GM. Perspectives in nutrition. 4th edition. Boston: WCB McGraw-Hill; 1999.
[2] Burke L, Heeley P. Dietary supplements and nutritional ergogenic aids in sport. In: Burke L, Deakin V, editors. Clinical sports nutrition. Sydney, Australia: McGraw-Hill Book Company; 1994. p. 227–84.
[3] Kimura N, Fukuwatari T, Sasaki R, et al. Vitamin intake in Japanese women college students. J Nutr Sci Vitaminol (Tokyo) 2003;49(3):149–55.
[4] Food and Nutrition Board of the Institute of Medicine. Dietary Reference Intakes for calcium, phosphorus, magnesium, vitamin D, and fluoride. Washington, DC: National Academy Press; 1997.
[5] Food and Nutrition Board of the Institute of Medicine. Dietary Reference intakes for thiamin, riboflavin, niacin, vitamin B6, folate, vitamin B12, pantothenic acid, biotin, and choline. Washington, DC: National Academy Press; 1998.
[6] Food and Nutrition Board of the Institute of Medicine. Dietary Reference Intakes for vitamin C, vitamin E, selenium, and carotenoids. Washington, DC: National Academy Press; 2000.
[7] Food and Nutrition Board of the Institute of Medicine. Dietary Reference Intakes for vitamin A, vitamin K, arsenic, boron, chromium, copper, iodine, iron, manganese, molybdenum, nickel, silicon, vanadium, and zinc. Washington, DC: National Academy Press; 2000.
[8] Food and Nutrition Board of the Institute of Medicine. Dietary Reference Intakes for water, potassium, sodium, chloride, and sulfate. Washington, DC: National Academy Press; 2005.
[9] Clark M, Reed DB, Crouse SF, et al. Pre- and post-season dietary intake, body composition, and performance indices of NCAA division I female soccer players. Int J Sport Nutr Exerc Metab 2003;13(3):303–19.
[10] Magkos F, Yannakoulia M. Methodology of dietary assessment in athletes: concepts and pitfalls. Curr Opin Clin Nutr Metab Care 2003;6(5):539–49.
[11] Leblanc JCh, Le Gall F, Grandjean V, et al. Nutritional intake of French soccer players at the Clairefontaine Training Centre. Int J Sport Nutr Exerc Metab 2002;12(3):268–80.
[12] Rico-Sanz J, Frontera WR, Mole PA, et al. Dietary and performance assessment of elite soccer players during a period of intense training. Int J Sport Nutr 1998;8(3):230–40.
[13] Iglesias-Gutierrez E, Garcia-Roves PM, Rodriguez C, et al. Food habits and nutritional status assessment of adolescent soccer players: a necessary and accurate approach. Can J Appl Physiol 2005;30(1):18–32.
[14] Ruiz F, Irazusta A, Gil S, et al. Nutritional intake in soccer players of different ages. J Sports Sci 2005;23(3):235–42.
[15] Paschoal VC, Amancio OM. Nutritional status of Brazilian elite swimmers. Int J Sport Nutr Exerc Metab 2004;14(1):81–94.
[16] Rankinen T, Lyytikainen S, Vanninen E, et al. Nutritional status of the Finnish elite ski jumpers. Med Sci Sports Exerc 1998;30(11):1592–7.
[17] Ziegler PJ, Jonnalagadda SS, Nelson JA, et al. Contribution of meals and snacks to nutrient intake of male and female elite figure skaters during peak competitive season. J Am Coll Nutr 2002;21(2):114–9.
[18] Hassapidou MN, Manstrantoni A. Dietary intakes of elite female athletes in Greece. J Hum Nutr Diet 2001;14(5):391–6.
[19] Papadopoulou SK, Papadopoulou SD, Gallos GK. Macro- and micro-nutrient intake of adolescent Greek female volleyball players. Int J Sport Nutr Exerc Metab 2002;12(1):73–80.

[20] Beals KA. Eating behaviors, nutritional status, and menstrual function in elite female adolescent volleyball players. J Am Diet Assoc 2002;102(9):1293–6.
[21] Kim SH, Kim HY, Kim WK, et al. Nutritional status, iron-deficiency-related indices, and immunity of female athletes. Nutrition 2002;18(1):86–90.
[22] Mullins VA, Houtkooper LB, Howell WH, et al. Nutritional status of US elite female heptathletes during training. Int J Sport Nutr Exerc Metab 2001;11(3):299–314.
[23] Gropper SS, Sorrels LM, Blessing D. Copper status of collegiate female athletes involved in different sports. Int J Sport Nutr Exerc Metab 2003;13(3):343–57.
[24] Gropper SS, Blessing D, Dunham K, et al. Iron status of female collegiate athletes involved in different sports. Biol Trace Elem Res 2006;109(1):1–14.
[25] Zhu YI, Haas JD. Iron depletion without anemia and physical performance in young women. Am J Clin Nutr 1997;66:334–41.
[26] Martinez-Torres C, Cubeddu L, Dillmann E, et al. Effect of exposure to low temperature on normal and iron-deficient subjects. J Physiol 1984;246:R380–3.
[27] Beard JL, Borel MJ, Derr J. Impaired thermoregulation and thyroid function in iron-deficiency anemia. Am J Clin Nutr 1990;52:13–9.
[28] Beard J, Tobin B, Green W. Evidence for thyroid hormone deficiency in iron-deficient anemic rats. J Nutr 1989;119:772–8.
[29] Rosenzweig PH, Volpe SL. Iron, thermoregulation, and metabolic rate. Crit Rev Food Sci Nutr 1999;39(2):131–48.
[30] Harris Rosenzweig P, Volpe SL. Effect of iron supplementation on thyroid hormone levels and resting metabolic rate in two college female athletes: a case study. Int J Sport Nutr Exerc Metab 2000;10(4):434–43.
[31] Lozoff B. Behavioral alterations in iron deficiency. Adv Pediatr 1988;35:331–59.
[32] Gleeson M, Nieman DC, Pedersen BK. Exercise, nutrition and immune function. J Sports Sci 2004;22(1):115–25.
[33] Petersen HL, Peterson CT, Reddy MB, et al. Body composition, dietary intake, and iron status of female collegiate swimmers and divers. Int J Sport Nutr Exerc Metab 2006;16(3):281–95.
[34] Beals KA, Manore MM. Nutritional status of female athletes with subclinical eating disorders. J Am Diet Assoc 1998;98(4):419–25.
[35] Janelle KC, Barr SI. Nutrient intakes and eating behavior sores of vegetarian and nonvegetarian women. J Am Diet Assoc 1995;95(2):180–6, 189.
[36] Ziegler P, Sharp R, Hughes V, et al. Nutritional status of teenage female competitive figure skaters. J Am Diet Assoc 2002;102(3):374–9.
[37] Ziegler PJ, Nelson JA, Jonnalagadda SS. Nutritional and physiological status of US national figure skaters. Int J Sport Nutr 1999;9(4):345–60.
[38] Jonnalagadda SS, Ziegler PJ, Nelson JA. Food preferences, dieting behaviors, and body image perceptions of elite figure skaters. Int J Sport Nutr Exerc Metab 2004;14(5): 594–606.
[39] Constantini NW, Eliakim A, Zigel L, et al. Iron status of highly active adolescents: evidence of depleted iron stores in gymnasts. Int J Sport Nutr Exerc Metab 2000;10(1):62–70.
[40] Dubnov G, Constantini NW. Prevalence of iron depletion and anemia in top-level basketball players. Int J Sport Nutr Exerc Metab 2004;14(1):30–7.
[41] Tsalis G, Nikolaidis MG, Mougios V. Effects of iron intake through food or supplement on iron status and performance of healthy adolescent swimmers during a training season. Int J Sports Med 2004;25(4):306–13.
[42] Vasankari T, Kujala U, Sarna S, et al. Effects of ascorbic acid and carbohydrate ingestion on exercise induced oxidative stress. J Sports Med Phys Fitness 1998;38(4):281–5.
[43] Bryant RJ, Ryder J, Martino P, et al. Effects of vitamin E and C supplementation either alone or in combination on exercise-induced lipid peroxidation in trained cyclists. J Strength Cond Res 2003;17(4):792–800.
[44] Peake JM. Vitamin C: effects of exercise and requirements with training. Int J Sport Nutr Exerc Metab 2003;13(2):125–51.

[45] Maughan R. The athlete's diet: nutritional goals and dietary strategies. Proc Nutr Soc 2002;61(1):87–96.
[46] Economos CD, Bortz SS, Nelson ME. Nutritional practices of elite athletes: practical recommendations. Sports Med 1993;16(6):381–99.
[47] American College of Sports Medicine, American Dietetic Association, Dietitians of Canada. Joint Position Statement: nutrition and athletic performance. American College of Sports Medicine, American Dietetic Association, Dietitians of Canada. Med Sci Sports Exerc 2000;32(12):2130–45.

Clin Sports Med 26 (2007) 131–135
CLINICS IN SPORTS MEDICINE
ELSEVIER SAUNDERS

INDEX

A

B

Note: Page numbers of article titles are in **boldface** type.

0278-5919/07/$ – see front matter
doi:10.1016/S0278-5919(06)00091-3
© 2007 Elsevier Inc. All rights reserved.
sportsmed.theclinics.com

Moving?

Make sure your subscription moves with you!

To notify us of your new address, find your **Clinics Account Number** (located on your mailing label above your name), and contact customer service at:

E-mail: elspcs@elsevier.com

800-654-2452 (subscribers in the U.S. & Canada)
407-345-4000 (subscribers outside of the U.S. & Canada)

Fax number: 407-363-9661

Elsevier Periodicals Customer Service
6277 Sea Harbor Drive
Orlando, FL 32887-4800

*To ensure uninterrupted delivery of your subscription, please notify us at least 4 weeks in advance of move.

ELSEVIER